Mind's Mission

Our vision is of a society that promotes and protects good mental health for all, and that treats people with experience of mental distress fairly, positively, and with respect.

The needs and experiences of people with mental distress drive our work and we make sure their voice is heard by those who influence change.

Our independence gives us the freedom to stand up and speak out on the real issues that affect daily lives.

We provide information and support, campaign to improve policy and attitudes and, in partnership with independent local Mind associations, develop local services.

We do all this to make it possible for people who experience mental distress to live full lives, and play their full part in society.

First published in the UK by
Mind
15-19 Broadway
Stratford
London E15 4BQ

Illustrations: Arvind Shah
Designed and typeset by Intertype, London
Printed and bound in the UK by Newnorth

ISBN: 1-903567-68-8

Note: The material contained in this book is set out in good faith for general guidance and no liability can be accepted for loss or expense incurred as a result of relying in particular circumstances on statements made in the book.

Moving on
from **depression**

Claire Rayner and
Elizabeth Spring

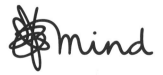

**For better
mental health**

Foreword

This book has been written for the very large number of people in this country affected by depression.

Every effort has been made to ensure that you will find answers to the questions people in this situation ask. That may sound a little boastful, but as someone who has experienced bouts of depression all her life, and who has been married for almost half a century to a man who suffers a much more severe form of it, I truly believe you will find what you seek in these pages.

It may sound absurd to say that this sometimes devastating condition can ever be beneficial, but I have to say that if I had not experienced depression, I might also never have experienced the most enjoyable, productive and therapeutic career that anyone could wish for.

This is partly because, like most people with a lifelong tendency to depression, I did not have it all the time. It first made itself known to me when I was about ten years old and hovering on the edge of puberty, which is known to be a trigger of hormone-induced depression in women. Thereafter, I had major episodes after the birth of each of my three children and around the menopause, and unfortunately am currently dealing with a non-hormonal, but still very common, form of depression as I learn to come to terms with old age.

I have been fortunate to have had my work as therapy, as well as the medication and time to talk my doctors provided. I found that when I sat down at my typewriter and started to write something – anything – the depression was pushed out of my mind by having to concentrate on the job.

During the times I was not burdened with misery, nagging guilt and the unbearably grey world I seemed to inhabit, I found the same techniques that helped me work when I was depressed seemed to flower into a creativity that continued when I was well. I wrote some of the novels with which I am most pleased during those times. The same has been true for my husband, an artist who has produced some of his most splendid work as he battled with his own demons.

Please believe me – there is light at the end of the tunnel.

Claire Rayner

Contents

Introduction

Welcome to this guide to surviving depression. You have taken the first step to getting help. This book is intended for people experiencing depression and for friends and relatives who want to find out how to help them. The information is based on what works for other people who have been through what you are feeling. The book is written for you and about you – there should be sections that you will find useful and you can skip the sections that don't apply to you. The information can then be built into a personal package for you to learn how to survive depression and move on from it.

Depression is the most common mental health problem in the UK. At its mildest, depression manifests itself in a persistent low mood and in physical tiredness, making the tasks of everyday life feel more difficult and less enjoyable or worthwhile. Major depression involves feelings of hopelessness and helplessness, at its most severe leading to suicidal thoughts and actions.

The symptoms of depression can include disturbed sleep or appetite, low energy or fatigue, loss of interest in sex, poor concentration, low mood, agitation, feelings of guilt and hopelessness, and the inability to derive interest or pleasure from activities you used to enjoy.

There is no one single cause of depression. Some people are more prone to depression than others for a range of possible reasons, including family background and painful past experience. Certain life events and social situations can trigger a depressive episode, lead to further deterioration or make recovery more difficult. These include physical illness, major life changes (such as moving house or retirement), poverty, isolation, bereavement, relationship breakdown and being the victim of a physical or sexual attack.

Help, advice and support

Many people liken depression to drowning in despair. People close to those who are depressed often feel they are also going under. This book is a safety line passing on the knowledge that there is help available – help that really does work.

Each chapter looks at a particular type of depression, life events that can trigger it or strategies for moving on. The book will give you ideas about how to find help, support and advice from the wide network of organisations and self-help groups, from health providers, books and the internet. There is a list of contacts at the end of the book. Depression can be overcome – it is important to remember that if one approach doesn't suit you, there are others you can try.

There are many triggers for depression and many types of people who experience it, so a wide range of treatments and approaches has been developed. Some help you cope, some change the chemical balances that affect mood, others focus on physical health or on talking and discovering patterns of thinking and feeling that started in childhood. Many people find that a combination of approaches provides the best treatment. Drugs, even the modern antidepressants (see page 51), have side effects and may not be desirable long term for cases of mild depression. They can, however, help you regain your balance long enough to try exercise, relaxation or meditation techniques, or one of the talking therapies such as cognitive behaviour therapy (see page 58).

This book looks at physical, emotional and circumstantial causes of depression and suggests practical ways of addressing them, both at home and with professional help and support. If something is not relevant to you, skip it and look for the information which you relate to. A big part of being depressed is the belief that nothing can help, that no one can make you feel better. Sometimes it feels as if the depressed reality is the only one you have ever known. Remind yourself of the times when you didn't feel this way and tell yourself the dark times will pass.

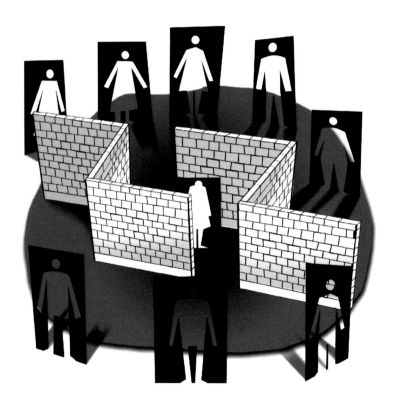

Chapter 1

What is depression?

Tens of millions of people in Britain experience depression at some stage in their lives. Some go through it once, others repeatedly. It can last for a few days as an after effect of flu or other viruses. For other people, the feelings can continue, without treatment, for months or even years. Such a wide-ranging experience obviously has an almost equally wide range of treatments and there are various schools of thought on what causes depression and how to help. The commonly accepted theories are:

1   Depression is a condition caused by chemical imbalances, which can be treated through drug therapy.

2   Depression is a learnt response to trauma or grief, which can be traced, talked through and moved on from.

3   Depression results from the repression of a painful emotion such as anger or sadness.

4   Depression is a combination of these factors, sometimes triggered by a bad experience, stress, tiredness or relationship breakdown.

5   The body holds on to distress by expressing it
    mentally as depression.

Sometimes people respond to a crisis or trauma by
becoming depressed. Then they get more depressed
because of waking up each day feeling so bad. The
original cause becomes lost and the depression feeds off
itself. Recognising these feelings, and getting help to
look at the original triggers, can help you escape from
the downward spiral.

I am going to list the most usual experiences of
depression. This will help break down what you or your
loved one are going through, so you can address any
feelings, physical symptoms, practical difficulties, social
situations, work and play as necessary.

Thoughts and feelings

Think about the following statements. Which of these
experiences is familiar to you?

1   You find it hard to sleep at night. You lie awake
    thinking negative thoughts for hours.

2   You are always tired and want to sleep all day.

3   You have lost interest in sex.

4   You have unexplained aches and pains.

5   You have no appetite – food may even make you
    feel sick.

6   You no longer take pleasure in activities you used to enjoy.

7   You are restless, can't sit still and find it hard to concentrate.

8   You are irritated and angry with friends, workmates and family.

9   You often think of suicide as a way out.

10 You have feelings of worthlessness or guilt.

11 You do not enjoy socialising, or you never go out.

12 You feel tearful and sad most of the time.

13 You cannot think of a way through.

14 You resent the way people try to help because they cannot understand you.

15 You put on a front, because you think nobody could bear the real you.

All these experiences are normal signs of depression. Do they relate to you or someone you're close to? If you answered that you feel several of these most of the time, and the feelings have lasted more than three or four weeks, it is important that you get in touch with a support organisation or your GP. There is a list of contacts at the back of the book.

Identifying the causes

Unhappiness is the normal response to events such as loss and illness, which most of us have to face in our lives. It will usually resolve itself with time and should not require medical treatment. Depression is when someone is stuck in this state and cannot move on.

Nowadays, with people living much more isolated lives than their forebears, the networks to help people get through bereavement, disappointment, loneliness and difficulties within families have often disappeared. Yet the long processes of grieving or starting along a new path after a significant life change are still necessary. A variety of helplines, mutual support groups and counselling sessions has been set up by people who have gone through difficult times to try to help others deal with their natural feelings of loss and sorrow.

Trained counsellors can help you identify why the depression started, and friends and family can then provide support. Neither you nor your immediate circle will have to deal with the condition alone. Samaritans will listen to you any time of the day or night. The list of organisations at the end of the book tells you about other people who will offer immediate help. People who have found ways to survive and move on from depression have set up self-help groups to pass on their expertise.

Antidepressants might help in the short term, too – when the physical and emotional symptoms are lifted, you can learn how to cope with the life events that are stressing you.

Depression can sometimes be caused by a physical condition. Mood is influenced by the thyroid gland, which controls your metabolic rate. An underactive thyroid (hypothyroidism) can cause depression. An underactive thyroid can usually be treated, and if you have other symptoms of this condition (such as weight gain, coarse dry hair, dry skin, hair loss or intolerance to cold) your doctor may suggest you take a blood test. In this case you won't get better by treating the depression, only by treating the underlying cause.

Depression may also come on very suddenly in response to certain foodstuffs or alcoholic drinks. As such reactions are very individual, they are very rarely recognised, so you may continue consuming the trigger item, while the problem gets worse and you cannot think what has caused it. If you identify the trigger, the depression usually lifts within 24 hours, so if you find you are suddenly depressed and have no life events that account for it, its worth looking at your recent diet to see if there is anything there that may be the culprit.

Trying to help someone with depression?

If you are a close friend or relative of someone living with depression, you may relate to some of the following statements as well:

1   You have tried and tried but the other person 'will not try'.
2   You are being taken over by the other person's negative attitude.
3   You feel angry and resentful a lot of the time.

4 You have needs as well but they are never acknowledged.

5 Your relationship has become that of a carer.

6 You feel guilty.

7 You do not know what to do.

8 You secretly want to escape.

9 You want someone else to come and take over for you.

These are all common feelings when you are close to someone who is depressed. They do not mean that you are uncaring. Sometimes acknowledging the feelings may be enough to help you through them, but more often they mean it is time for you both to find outside help. One close relative described her experience as "passing a parcel of pain backwards and forwards between us, neither wanting to be left with it". It is not a sign of failure that you cannot cope alone.

If more than three statements from the list apply to you, it might mean you are doing too much by yourself. You need to prioritise finding support for yourself. Professionals have supervision and support to do their work, so why shouldn't you?

The mental health charity Mind has a network of affiliated organisations throughout England and Wales, which often offer support to carers. Couple counselling, contacting a helpline such as Mind*info*Line or

Samaritans, or an honest confidential talk to a trusted friend can all help.

What partners, friends and family can do to help

When you are feeling worthless, ugly, hateful, hollow and scared, being expected to 'pull yourself together' is about as helpful as asking someone with a sprained ankle to forget it and come out for a run.

It is useful to offer comfort, without dismissing the person's experience. It may look to a friend or carer that the person with depression is wallowing in or clinging on to negativity. Indeed, many depressed people talk as if they have a mission to convert everyone else to an awareness of all the hopeless horrors of the world. They are not doing this deliberately. Depression distorts how we interpret what goes on around us. It may help to listen and agree that the friend's experience is truly horrible. Many people long to know that their relatives or friends can acknowledge their feelings without being overwhelmed by depression as well. Consciously trying this – listening without giving advice or arguing – can often help directly. Sometimes, however, this is too uncomfortable. The carer can be so distressed by what is happening to their friend that they desperately need them to stop sharing their feelings.

This is not wrong.

Without professional training, very few people are able to keep on listening to despair, bitterness and pain day after day. If the person experiencing depression cannot bear themselves, they may be unconsciously trying to prove that you cannot bear them either. Reassure them that you care, but that you need help to help them. GPs see patients with depression every day. Go together, or go separately, because nobody will judge either of you for asking for outside help with this.

Isolation

Many couples, where one or both experience depression, find themselves gradually becoming isolated from the wider world. Friends disappear, possibly feeling helpless or overwhelmed. It becomes more difficult to face a social life and shared activities seem irrelevant or too much effort. Sometimes one partner begins to stay at work late, or takes up an activity the other does not want to share. Home turns into the place where everything focuses on depression, gloom and despair.

Single people often become isolated too, turning inwards and never wanting to go out, phone friends or accept invitations. When the invitations peter out, this can seem to prove that nobody cares.

It can help to plan a few small practical steps to begin to change this pattern of loneliness. At first, a person with depression will not feel like going out socially, however lonely they are, but beginning to address some of the symptoms of depression does work for lots of people. Briefly, the thinking is that if we deliberately short-circuit familiar, negative habits, then the feelings attached to them change too. Starting very gently, with realistic goals, will lead to slow achievable changes.

Loss of libido

It has been said that the most important sexual organ is the brain. Depression is often accompanied by a decreased sex drive and some commonly prescribed antidepressants can have the side effect of lowering libido or even causing temporary erectile dysfunction. This may put even more pressure on a relationship at a time when the person experiencing depression has most need of their partner.

It's important for partners to understand that loss of libido is a symptom of depression which can lead to further stress, guilt and feelings of isolation.

If you think a lack of interest in sex is caused by drugs you have been prescribed to treat depression, discuss it with your GP. Maybe another antidepressant won't have this side effect, or they might advise taking a short break from the medication.

Short-term goals

It is useless to tell a person experiencing depression to "pull themselves together", because they would get out of the state if they could. The miseries of depression are devastating; no one would tolerate these feelings out of any sort of idleness. Moving on is not just a matter of will-power after depression has taken hold. The next stage is therefore about starting to take control of everyday behaviour, not trying to find a quick fix.

When someone is depressed, all the pleasure in life is dimmed or absent. It can even be difficult to acknowledge that anything, ever, gives happiness. Yet an extraordinary moment of light can happen through something very simple, such as coming across a sunlit tree in the park, having a friendly exchange in the cornershop, or relaxing with a bath or walk. It is really important to keep sight of the outside world. So think of some short-term goals, actions that are small, realistic and can take place over the next few hours.

What sort of goals?

These suggestions work both for the person who feels depressed and for partners and close friends. Please just try one and keep it small. Or think of a goal of your own.

Thinking of it is today's goal – try it out later, or tomorrow.

Staying in bed all day?	Take a shower or shave when you first get up – if you keep up your personal appearance you will feel better about yourself.
Not eating or only eating junk food?	Have something tasty, healthy and easy, like a piece of fruit.
Angry all the time?	Write it down, or even make a drawing – just for yourself.
Feeling closed in?	Go for a short walk; even if it's just to the newsagents.
Home is a mess?	Change your bedclothes and put the dirty linen in the wash.
Overwhelmed?	Lie on the floor for five minutes and breathe deeply, arms and hands relaxing more with each outward breath.
Not sleeping?	Try a short walk to help your body relax.

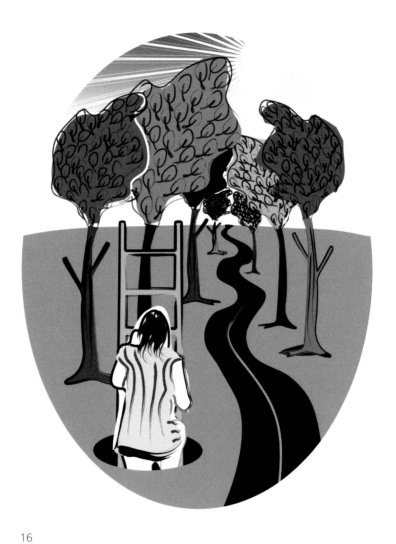

Chapter 2

Looking after yourself

When you are experiencing depression or are living with someone who is really down, it is more important than ever to treat yourself with care and kindness.

Try to make time for activities that are relaxing, enjoyable. Socialising, going to a film or other outside event, having a couple of hours in the library or art gallery, arranging a short evening class where you can enjoy a hobby or pursue an ambition, will all help you rediscover a part of yourself which may be temporarily lost. Swimming, walking, yoga or any form of low-key exercise will help you unwind. These will all help friends or partners too, as everything will no longer centre on depression.

Life does not have to be a constant grind of unhappiness because one of you feels so bad. It is not hard-hearted to enjoy a short evening out with other friends, or a denial of depression to take a walk in the park.

Comfort

Many people experiencing depression find it very hard to acknowledge that anything is ever pleasant. This is hard work for them and for their friends. So plan in some time apart to give each other a little breathing space. During this time, read a book, take a long bath, go for a swim, work in the garden or meet up with friends. The idea is to do something small and enjoyable, not to tackle a major task that might get left unfinished; so keep it simple.

It is not a partner's fault that someone feels depressed, just as it is not the person's fault that his or her worldview is so bleak. Look after yourselves as two separate individuals, and plan a regular morning, evening or weekend time for this. Life does not have to stop when someone experiences depression. You may each resent the other if everything centres on the depression, and it is vital to plan in other elements to your time.

Rebalancing your diet and beginning to take exercise help the process of recovery. Alongside talking to a trusted professional and your friends, you can slowly rebuild your physical and emotional systems as the depression ebbs away.

Time-out for carers

Unless you find time to look after your own needs, you are likely to become overwhelmed. This can be helped.

• Having a pleasant time yourself does not take anything away from the person you are supporting.

- No one is being realistic if they expect you to be superhuman, including yourself. You could be doing more than is possible for one person alone.

- There are plenty of places to find help with this situation.

- It is a sign of courage and good sense to accept such support.

- People around you may well accept everything you offer without seeing how tired you are. If you keep offering, you need somewhere to refuel your own emotional resources.

Take five minutes now to think about a realistic, achievable activity that gives you pleasure. It can be anything – reading a book, washing the car, watching a favourite soap, listening to music, or climbing a hill to take in the view and put the world in perspective.

Write your chosen activity here:

When did you last do this?

If the activity is one that you want to do but keep putting off, is it possible to plan it this week?

If so, make a date now and come back and tick it off when you've done it.

If it is not realistic to do it at present, what could you do instead?

Make it something that would be possible for you to do and set a date.

Write it here:

Deserving happiness

Many people with depression have had repeated experiences in their lives which end up giving them the idea that they do not deserve happiness.

Carers may also often have had childhoods where they were not cared for, or had to learn how to look after parents whose own difficulties made it impossible for them to give proper care to their children. Finding a career, partner or friends whose needs enable you to continue playing a supportive giving role can feel deeply right and familiar to you. However, even if you are very good at making others feel better, that does not satisfy your own need to be looked after sometimes too.

If this applies to you, you're probably very good at seeing how to help other people. Accepting that there is a place for healthy, enjoyable selfishness in your life can be something people have to deliberately think about, acknowledge and learn.

The short-term goals mentioned at the beginning of the chapter can be the first steps towards this. Please think of one now. Begin by acknowledging the fact that you deserve it:

Other people

Friends and extended families often disappear when someone experiences depression for longer than a couple of weeks. Depression is annoying, frightening and demoralising both to experience and to be near. It doesn't mean that people are uncaring – they often just don't know what to do. In big cities, as well as in isolated rural areas, people frequently don't know their neighbours and live away from their relatives. This tends to reinforce the self-imposed isolation, which is often a feature of depression.

Major life events like having a baby, going through bereavement, children growing up and leaving home, or periods of unemployment used to involve community rituals and practical neighbourly responses. Single parents, many of whom are unsupported, now head a quarter of families. We are offered media images of ideal families with glamorous parents surrounded by beautiful children, which make the great majority of people who don't live like that feel there's something out there they can't ever attain. On the other hand, watching the news makes us aware of every tragedy and cruelty around the globe like never before.

Not surprisingly, when a person feels raw and horribly open to all this, they tell everyone about it insistently. Many people react by staying away and the person experiencing depression and their family can feel more and more alone.

There are usually one or two people who continue to offer time and a listening ear. Unfortunately, they can end up being an audience to stories about how uncaring everyone else is. This stops the person with depression acknowledging the good things they are doing and adds to their bleak view of the outside world.

Friends

If some friends do not feel able to share the pain of depression, this does not mean they are uncaring. Cutting off from them completely may mean that you miss out on the good things you share.

Others may not realise that you are disappointed with them. We all misunderstand each other sometimes. If you can do it in a clear, friendly way it might be worth gently checking out why people are not in touch. They may be going through a hard time of their own, have experienced your situation themselves and don't want to be reminded of it at the moment, or just not realise that you are so unhappy. Have you asked them directly? If they are very important to you, can you leave it for a while then suggest something you can do together?

Not everyone likes intense emotional sessions, but if you have a good underlying friendship it is probably worth trying to make contact for some undemanding social activity. You can talk it all through much later when the time feels right.

It is common to feel that people are asking too much and therefore to retreat and give nothing rather than offering a little. For example, if a single parent is despairing because they never go out, the friend may not offer to help because they don't want to end up baby-sitting every week. They may not realise that even once would be wonderful.

People sometimes shy away from those undergoing bereavement and relationship breakdown because they are so uncomfortable with this level of grief. This is a normal response and does not mean either the friend or the bereaved person is wrong, but it can be extremely hurtful.

Someone else may not be able to come up with a solution to the world's problems and thinks offering to go to the pub would be ridiculous. Feeling guilty about not helping is so unpleasant that they may stay away and then the vicious circle starts. So the single parent stops having visits as well as not going out, and the depressed person in anguish about the state of the world is personally lonely too.

Can you think of a small gesture which opens the door to friendship again? This is not to devalue your feeling of betrayal, but does put it into the context of the longer view of your friendships. Next time someone rings you up or sees you in the street, deliberately ask them a couple of questions about themselves, keep it light and praise yourself afterwards for succeeding.

If that seems too much for you to do at the moment, then practise being friendly with the person selling newspapers or the supermarket checkout worker. Tiny human interactions are really helpful to regain a sense of how many nice people there are about. You relearn that you do not frighten people away and that this stage of your life is temporary – you *will* feel better.

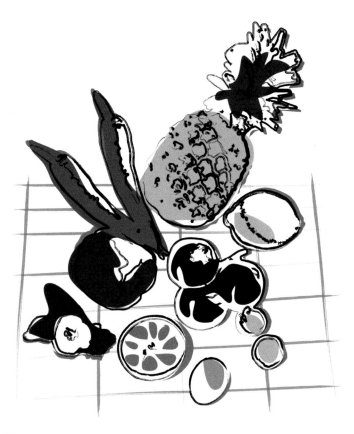

Lifestyle

There are many explanations for the cause-and-effect relationship between food and drink and mood. The following are some examples:

Fluctuations in blood sugar levels are associated with changes in mood and energy, and are affected by what we eat.

Chemicals in the brain influence the way we think, feel and behave. They can be affected by what we've eaten.

It's generally accepted that how we feel can influence what we choose to eat or drink. What is less well known is how what we eat can affect our mental functioning. The use of caffeine is one example of what is a complex relationship. Caffeine, found in tea, coffee, cola drinks and chocolate, is probably the most widely used behaviour-modifying drug in the world. We often choose to drink it if we are feeling tired and irritable, because it can give us a boost and help us to concentrate. Having a cup of coffee or tea also has a lot of positive psychological associations. We meet a friend for 'coffee and a chat' or give ourselves a break by sitting down with a cup of tea, and these things are very important. But too much caffeine (which is a different amount for each of us) can cause symptoms such as anxiety, nervousness and depression.

Appetite

Many people find they cannot eat when they are severely depressed. The sight or thought of food makes them feel sick. They get a knot in the stomach or throat when food is in front of them or just never have an appetite.

We all need to eat to stay healthy and when your blood sugar is lowered depression gets worse. If you are feeling down to start off with, starving yourself makes it much harder to begin to feel better.

Losing your appetite can start when a relationship suddenly breaks down, you experience bereavement or some other terrible shock. The reflex to curl up is natural and can do no harm for a day or two. After that, you need to gently coax yourself to eat or drink or you will become ill. Sometimes only chocolate or other childhood comfort food seems edible. That's fine for a short while, but you also need to begin to take in small regular amounts of carbohydrates or you will become dizzy and weak. You do not need that on top of feeling so bad, and prolonged avoidance of food will mean you are unable to deal with anything. If you feel disgusted by food, try taking fluids to begin with. This can be a simple fruit juice or smoothie.

All the traditional foods are healthy and comforting. A couple of mouthfuls of a protein and carbohydrate meal will warm you and stop the shakiness caused by not eating. Pasta with tomato-based sauces, shepherd's pie, lentil dhal and rice, baked potato with some grilled meat or vegetarian sausages, baked beans, cheese on toast, apple crumble and custard, can all be prepared very simply and initially eaten in tiny portions to whet the appetite.

Comfort eating

Sometimes food becomes the ultimate comfort for someone who is depressed and this can bring its own problems. It feels as if the only way to escape the physical pain and hollowness of depression is to eat. Many convenience foods like cake, burgers, chips and pies are deeply satisfying because they give instant comfort. Often the meals that seem to make you feel better are the ones to slowly cut down if they are all you ever want. It is a difficult pattern to change.

Body image is a central part of who we are, like it or not. Becoming heavily overweight is a health risk in itself, but if it is a result of depressed overeating, then a vicious circle is set up. You don't like how you are living or how you look, so you turn to the biscuit tin, ice cream carton or pizza box to feel better. The worse you feel about doing this, the more you want to. It is not a sign of weak will to become dependent on food.

We learn our eating habits in childhood, so if you have always been given sweets or puddings as a reward or treat, naturally that will remain a comfort when you are older. Studies have also shown a genetic link to obesity. So if these factors are combined, you have to learn a new relationship with eating. Slowly you can begin to enjoy food without using it to control unhappiness or depression.

There is lots of professional support available for this. GPs, counsellors and community nurses can all help.

This is not a suggestion to go on a diet. If you are depressed, you don't want to feel worse by cutting out what comforts you. It is much more useful to start by finding new ways of getting comfort.

Does this relate to you? Maybe it would help to look at how you currently eat. Try jotting down what you eat today, including when, where and why. Think about these questions:

- Which foods do you eat most of?
- Do you continue eating even after you are full or have stopped enjoying the meal?
- Could you talk about changing your way of eating, or does this panic you?

What could you do instead?

Perhaps you might start by talking about food with a counsellor. Many people turn to eating instead of asking people to listen when they are feeling depressed. Food becomes a major problem as well as an answer to stress or loneliness. Pizzas are bad listeners – turn to your GP, a friend or counsellor instead.

Looking at what happened to start you overeating can untangle the associations with food, depression and comfort. When these are separated, food can become a way of nourishing yourself to have a fitter, healthier body. Comfort can be gained from activities that make you feel good about yourself. The causes of the depression or poor self-image can be looked at without being hidden by eating and consequent guilt or self-dislike.

You can slowly change your eating habits to enjoy more varieties of food. The links between poor diet and depression are well reported. However, it is not easy to suddenly change and still gain comfort and pleasure from a new regimen. A medical dietician can show you how to approach this and monitor your progress. They are not there to turn you into a movie star, but to support you step by step into becoming healthier.

A good way to start is to choose a delicious comforting food that is also 'healthy'. Your food should be a pleasure, not a guilty secret or a diet so boring it feels like a punishment. Plan one meal today which you will be pleased to have eaten afterwards. Food can be good for you and a comfort as well.

It can be a slow business finding other ways to have treats and look after yourself. Combining a gentle increase in exercise with a steady controlled change in your eating habits is the best and most effective way to begin. The next chapter describes simple effective relaxation techniques. These can also be treats in themselves and lead to a beneficial cycle of feeling more in control when stress hits you.

Alcohol

Alcohol is a commonly used and socially acceptable mood-altering drug. It is also implicated in some of our society's most entrenched problems such as violence and ill health.

While we may have a drink to relax after a hard day, it should be remembered that alcohol is a depressant. It can bring short-term relief from the symptoms of depression, but long term will only make them worse and does nothing to change the underlying causes. In fact it may well become one of them. If you regularly drink because you're unhappy – because of relationship problems, stress at work, or any of the other circumstances discussed in this book, you will only make things worse.

While most drinkers manage perfectly well, regular, heavy users can become tolerant and even addicted to alcohol in a way that can be hard to break. Addicts may use alcohol much like heroin, as a refuge from life, or as a means of facing what would otherwise seem unfaceable. It lowers people's inhibitions and encourages them to express their inner feelings, which may be aggression and frustration that emerge in violence.

Alcohol is the most toxic, or poisonous, of the commonly used non-medical drugs. Withdrawal causes sweating, anxiety, trembling and delirium. As with other addictions, escape is possible if the person is determined and, usually, if they are prepared to deal with other contributory personal issues.

Using drugs may bring underlying mental health problems to the surface, reinforce or worsen them. But it's very hard to tell cause from effect in these situations. Anybody who takes non-medical drugs may be trying, to some extent, to medicate themselves. Think about other ways to unwind; the next chapter explores simple and healthy ways to relieve stress.

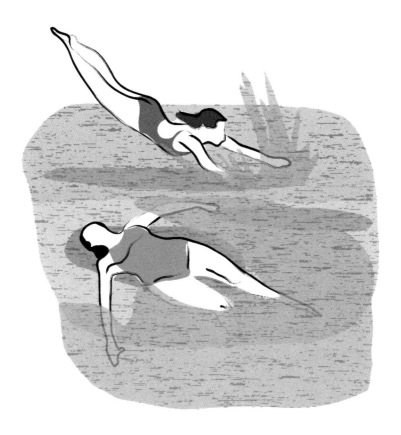

Body and mind: exercise and relaxation

Chapter 4

Relaxation techniques

One of the most effective relaxation techniques needs nothing but a quiet room, a couple of pillows and ten minutes of your time. Use music too if you like, or just listen to the rhythm of your own breathing. Friends and partners can take turns to talk the technique through for each other on consecutive evenings. It is effective by yourself, too. If you are doing the exercise alone, read it through twice before you start. If you're offering to help someone else, read it slowly and calmly out loud, leaving a couple of seconds between each sentence.

Put on some quiet music and make sure the room is warm before you start.

Controlled breathing

Find two pillows and lie down on a bed or the floor with one pillow below your knees and the other under your neck and head. ▶

Keep your hands and arms at your sides with the palms turned up. Let your tongue relax against the roof of your mouth and gently close your eyes.

This position means you are completely safe and supported, so you can begin to let your body relax and sink downwards with each outward breath.

Breathe slowly in to the count of five.

Breathe out and let your arms and hands sink down into the safe, warm, supporting surface below you.

Breathe in. You are controlling your own breathing, you are completely supported, let your arms become heavier and warmer with each outward breath.

Be aware of your shoulders. They have no weight to carry, you are lying safe and supported, and your head and neck are supported. As you breathe out, let your shoulders and arms and hands become heavier and warmer.

Breathe deeply in and let your shoulders and arms and hands relax and become warmer and heavier with each outward breath.

Pause and listen to the music. Using the rhythm of the music, let your breathing stay deep and even, deep and even. Feel your shoulders and hands and arms, warm and heavy.   ▶

Fill your mind with the rhythm and slowly breathe deeply in and then out.

Now you can lie for a couple of minutes noticing how your shoulders, arms and hands are resting supported and heavy.

Slowly open your eyes. Yawn, stretch and slowly, at your own pace, sit up.

This technique can be learnt then extended down the whole body over the course of half an hour.

Recognising where you are tense is a good way to start consciously relaxing in stressful situations.

At work or socially, you can consciously let your hands and shoulders relax while breathing out, without anyone noticing. Releasing the tension stops you getting wound up and helps you get in control of your feelings.

Practice for ten minutes every evening, or first thing when you wake up. After a while you will be able to empty your mind of everything but the music and the breathing rhythm, which can be a great relief.

Try to use this as one of your daily treats. It helps both someone who is depressed and their carer or partner. If you do it in the morning, follow up with fruit juice or an apple or orange, to bring up your blood sugar while your body is still relaxed. That will start your day with a little more energy to help you through the morning.

Meditation technique

Sit in a comfortable chair or propped up on pillows on your bed.

Think of your favourite colour.

Breathe deeply in and out three times, ensuring your whole chest fills as you breathe in.

Breathe deeply out right through to your belly with each outward breath.

Then, as you breathe in, fill your mind with the name of your favourite colour.

As you breathe out, visualise something peaceful in that colour: the sky, the sea, a sunset, a flower, a field, a forest – whatever you like.

Concentrate on the colour with each deep, even breath.

Try this for ten rhythmic breaths to start off with.

As other thoughts enter your mind, acknowledge them and let them go, replacing them with your colour.

Whenever you begin to feel stressed, think of the colour, and take three deep breaths to help you relax.

Exercise

Regular exercise, involving movement and deep breathing, will make you stronger, fitter and more confident, while teaching you effective, long-lasting ways to deeply relax. You can then deal with stress more successfully.

If you are physically unable to relax, think about trying a class in massage, yoga or t'ai chi. If you are caught in feelings of anger and you are reasonably fit, consider kickboxing. Beginners' classes have women and men of all ages and levels of fitness in them. Your GP may be able to advise you on a local exercise class specifically for people who need a gentle introduction. T'ai chi and yoga classes are available at beginners' level at local sports and community centres and suit all levels of fitness. They use breathing and very slow gentle movement to gradually build up strength and fitness.

Remember that however stressful your situation, it will not last forever. Depression can be a response to trauma or to feeling trapped. The first step out of it is to begin to find help to take control of your own responses to stress.

Can exercise improve your mood?

Studies of people from all age groups have shown the benefits of regular exercise in reducing symptoms of stress, depression and anxiety.

A brisk walk three times a week significantly reduces anxiety and helps with recovery from depression.

A study in 2000 (Babyak, M A et al., *Psychosomatic Medicine*) of 156 people with clinical depression showed the group of people who were treated through attending exercise classes had twice the recovery rate of those treated with just medication. The benefits continued after six months.

How does it work?

- Exercise increases your heart rate and relieves muscle tension.

- Sleep and appetite improve.

- As you become physically stronger, the feelings of apathy and tiredness recede.

- This enables you to cope with daily life and to be more objective when faced with problems.

- Self-esteem rises as you become fitter.

- You know you are responsible for your improvement and gain some control over your improved mood.

- You are concentrating on getting better rather than on what is wrong.

- Pushing yourself physically or taking out rage on a pillow or punch bag, rather than on partners or colleagues, can relieve feelings of anger and irritation.

- Endorphins, the body's own 'feel good' chemical, are produced after exercise and give a natural high.

- All the side effects of exercise are positive so you start a positive cycle, which you can control.

- You need daylight to produce vitamin D and feel well. Walking is free, does you good and can be done at any time.

Social benefits

Both someone living with depression and their partner or carer can benefit from taking regular exercise.

Withdrawal from society is a common symptom of depression. An exercise class has the activity as its focus, rather than socialising, so you can meet new people very gently, at a pace you choose, while becoming stronger and fitter. If you are not up to taking a class, then start moving by taking a book or magazine to a local park. The walk will do you good and the reading material gives you another focus when you get there.

Gardening is such a good form of exercise that some groups run 'green therapy' for people experiencing long-term mental health problems. The combination of being in touch with the earth, stretching, moving and being outside reaps huge benefits.

Joining a walking group is another non-threatening way to extend your social group. If you don't want to socialise, you can just walk. If there are potential friends there, so much the better.

A personal experience

Mary is 39, with two small children. Two years ago her life turned upside down with a series of tragedies, including bereavement, separation from her husband and the birth of a child with serious health problems. She hid away and spent much of her time crying and comfort eating. She became increasingly isolated. People stopped calling round and her weight mushroomed, making her self-conscious about going out.

She joined a swimming group and, with encouragement from her family, she carried on going to it. She is now a regular user of the local gym:

I wanted to be somewhere I didn't know anyone so they wouldn't know about all the dramas I'd been through.

I was flabby and overweight so it was good to be with other women who weren't too fit. It was actually a laugh, as well as making me see how out of condition I was.

I joined the gym with my sister. I give myself fitness goals to reach, to keep myself going back. Partly, it is a relief to concentrate on my body – not on all the sad thoughts going round and round.

It is good for the children to get out, even if it's only to the crèche.

I do feel better about myself now I am fitter. I am sleeping better and eating less rubbish.

I have contacted a bereavement counselling self-help group and see someone once a week who's been through my experience. The exercise gives me something to go out for and the counsellor helps me get through being at home.

I don't know why exercising is so helpful, but I know I feel so much better when I have been and that makes me go back and gives me something to look forward to.

Of course, one of the symptoms of depression is a deep reluctance to move or even get out of bed, let alone exercise.

Don't go from taking no exercise to full workouts. Remember the way to move on from depression is to take small steps that help you build on each success:

• Start really gently by stretching when you first get up.

• Walk slightly faster than usual when you move about at home.

• Ease yourself into exercising, by going one shop further than necessary to buy milk and bread, or by going up the stairs faster than usual.

• If you miss a day, it is easy to start again the next day.

The benefits start immediately and accumulate the more you do. However gently you start, exercise will make you feel better. You are giving yourself one of the best possible therapies and it is free and one which is available to everyone.

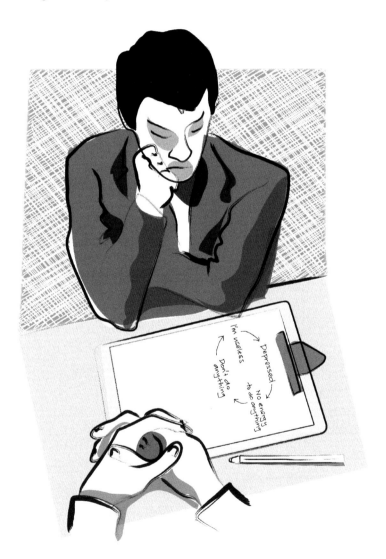

Triggers for depression and treatment options

Everyone has a variety of inner voices telling them how to make sense of their lives. Some therapies call this a script, and a script can be rewritten. People experiencing depression often have a script that tells a story of blame:

It is their own fault that they feel bad. No one has ever liked them or helped them – but how could they like or help someone so useless?

Everyone else is at fault. They don't care enough, don't understand and give stupid advice.

A person with depression feels small, helpless and despairing in a world where nobody cares. Yet it is possible to acknowledge these feelings and find ways to counter them.

Blame and guilt are powerful agents of depression because they help people deny any possibility of change. Although this is a terrible place to be, it is also, in some ways, safer than acknowledging the sadness and rage which underlie depression. It may be instinctive to take time out to heal after a shock, bereavement or unwanted life change. Withdrawing – to minimise the chance of further hurt – is another common mechanism of depression. But when it goes on for long enough to overshadow everything else, and prevents enjoyment of everyday pleasures, it is time to find ways of moving on.

Talking therapies can help people rewrite these scripts, but the process requires active participation and engagement.

Repetition

One symptom of depression can be the internal repetition of phrases, memories or events. Round and round go the same thoughts, during the day, in the middle of the night, drowning out everything that is happening around you.

A useful technique is to consciously interrupt these thoughts with something else:

1 Firstly, identify the nagging thoughts.

2 What triggers them?

3 How often do you go over them?

4 Picture your thoughts as a cassette tape, which can be switched on and off. Some people choose a time of day to let the 'tape' come on for 15 minutes, timing it with an alarm clock to make sure they switch it off again. The 15 minutes is used for a good wallow, then switch off and it's time to cook or go for a walk, concentrate on a book, ring someone or turn on the TV or radio.

5   Others find it better to learn how to turn the tape off every time it starts. As soon as the internal tape starts – actively interrupt it with something else.

6   Plan how to consciously interrupt patterns of negative thought. With a brisk NO? A deliberate turning to another train of thoughts? An activity? What would work for you?

7   It takes practice for this technique to work. Our brains follow set patterns and when a train of thought begins it needs conscious re-routing to change it.

8   Using a diary also helps. Write down ideas, plans, poetry and things you've noticed or enjoyed. Reading this back every couple of weeks shows you when you are caught in repetition, and what else is happening for you to build on.

Coping with long-term depression is a learnt skill. The most important part of it is to build on the elements of your life and personality that are not depressed. If these are not present at the moment, then set up a series of small, gentle journeys to find ways of bringing in some enjoyment. This will slowly create routes out of the persistent feelings and establish a strengthening experience of pleasure and hope.

Long-term depression

People who have lived with depression for a long time can become so used to the condition that it seems as if there is no other way of existing. This is exhausting for them and for those around them.

Depression is self-feeding. The longer it goes on, the more remote any other way of feeling becomes. There is a form of safety in this as well, because the early triggers for the onset of depression are lost within the physical and emotional fog of the condition. However, it is possible to allow yourself to slowly appreciate the balance of good and bad experiences available to everyone.

Many people learn coping techniques for being constantly depressed. These include:

1   Using a notebook to jot down daily notes of anything pleasurable or happy, to slowly build up a list of good experiences to remember and contemplate.

2   Building relationships with a support group or regularly using a helpline to keep the depression within one part of their lives.

3   Learning a system such as cognitive behaviour therapy to rethink how to approach day-to-day life and take charge of responses to it. Find out more on page 58.

4   Building on good experiences by repeating them and not dwelling on bad ones.

5 Feeling low but still getting up and moving through the day anyway.

6 Being very careful of yourself and deliberately choosing activities that involve going out into pleasant and undemanding environments.

7 Choosing healthy foods, which do not add to sugar-induced mood swings.

8 Avoiding unnecessary stress.

9 Telling people when you feel fragile and asking for consideration.

10 Being creative, either by making or listening to music, painting, drawing, writing and going to places where arts are exhibited or performed.

It may be useful to look at the following short questionnaire and see how to manage some aspects of this bout of depression.

When did the depression start?

What did you do at this time?

Did it help?

What can sometimes help you to feel better now?

What hinders?

How would you advise someone else in a similar situation?

Make a list of three things that you are currently missing through being depressed. These can be anything, but may include enjoyment, social life, trust, sex, ability to earn money, family intimacy, eating well or going out.

1

2

3

When it is impossible to listen to other people's suggestions, it can be hugely helpful to listen to your own – how would you advise someone else to address these issues?

Treatment

Whether it is through therapy, a support group, prescribed or alternative medication, or a strategy of exercise, counselling and goal setting, there is a route forward. It may be a combination of these things. Much research has shown that many highly creative people live with depression as the downside of their talent. Millions of people live with depression at some point in their lives, yet they do not all feel like this all the time. It is vital to allow the possibility that pleasure and enjoyment can return and that you can use your body and mind to get there.

There are many therapies available to people suffering depression. Different approaches suit different people. It is important to do some research and shop around for what works for you. Some people relax by exercising and others by taking a long bath. Some have a sweet tooth and others a savoury one. Similarly different schools of therapy suit different people.

Many practitioners suggest using medication in combination with talking therapy to get through a crisis or a particularly tough patch. While talking therapies may not produce results as quickly as drugs, they are free of physical side effects and appear to help prevent depression from recurring. GPs and patients may be tempted by the quick fix of antidepressants since there are currently long waiting lists for talking therapies on the NHS, and because these therapies require time and effort when compared with remembering to take medication. There has been a traditional split in the treatment of depression of mind vs brain – psychotherapy (talking therapies) vs psychopharmacology (drugs). However, there is strong evidence that antidepressants and psychotherapy produce similar changes in brain chemistry via different routes.

Antidepressants can start the healing process

While modern drugs are ever more sophisticated and targeted to specific functions of the brain, they still represent a somewhat scattergun approach to treating depression. Antidepressants work by increasing the activity and levels of chemicals produced naturally in the brain, which are thought to be suppressed during periods of depression. Knowledge of brain chemistry is still very limited and all antidepressants have other effects than those desired. Sometimes these unwanted effects can even increase certain symptoms of depression such as loss of libido or appetite. When deciding to use medication it is important to discuss this thoroughly with your doctor.

There are several different types of antidepressant, including:

- selective serotonin reuptake inhibitors (SSRIs)
- tricyclic antidepressants and
- monoamine oxidase inhibitors.

Side effects

The most common side effects associated with antidepressants include gastric upset (such as nausea), headaches, restlessness, anxiety, sleep disturbance and sexual difficulties. Such problems may be treatable by lowering the dose, changing to an alternative drug or stopping the drug for a while. There have also been reports in the press associating suicides and incidents when people have become uncharacteristically violent with their use of SSRIs.

You can find more details about side effects in the Mind booklet *Making sense of antidepressants,* which you can read on the Mind website www.mind.org.uk or order in print by writing to Mind Publications, 15-19 Broadway, London E15 4BQ or ringing 0844 448 4448.

A good doctor will carefully tailor the prescription to suit you and your condition, and monitor your progress and any side effects. You may have to try different drugs to find the antidepressant or combination of drugs that works best for you.

SSRIs and young people

None of these drugs has ever been licensed for anyone under the age of 18, but they have been widely prescribed. Research suggests that SSRIs are not effective in this age group and are more prone to cause side effects, including suicidal feelings, in young people than in adults. The government agency responsible for regulating the use of prescription drugs published guidance in 2003 that no SSRIs should be given to this age group except on the advice of a child psychiatrist.

Coming off antidepressants

Withdrawal or 'discontinuation' reactions can occur with all major types of antidepressant. Problems are more likely to occur after abrupt withdrawal and longer courses of treatment. Reactions usually start suddenly within a few days of stopping the antidepressant (or, less commonly, of reducing its dose) and usually disappear within one day to three weeks.

The probability of withdrawal problems and the symptoms vary depending on the type of antidepressant. Common symptoms include gastric problems, loss of appetite, sleep disturbance, headaches, mood changes and restlessness. With SSRIs the commonest symptoms appear to be dizziness, light-headedness, numbness, tingling and sensations that resemble having electric shocks. In a minority of people discontinuation reactions are severe and very troublesome.

The British National Formulary (BNF) provides UK healthcare professionals with information on the selection and use of medicines. It recommends that if antidepressants have been prescribed continuously for eight weeks or more they should not be stopped abruptly, but should be reduced gradually over four weeks. Some reports suggest that tapering off the dose may not be necessary when switching between SSRIs. If discontinuation reactions are severe, the antidepressant may need to be restarted and the dose tapered off very gradually. For some people who experience major problems, however, this advice may be inadequate. Mind has published a report *Coping with come off* which details the experiences of people trying to come off psychiatric drugs and is available from Mind Publications, 15-19 Broadway, London E15 4BQ, telephone 0844 448 4448.

St John's wort

The herbal remedy St John's wort is effective for many people with mild to medium depression. It is available from chemists and health food shops as a tablet or tincture. It's worth remembering, however, that many standard medicines are based on plant extracts, and just because something is a herb doesn't mean that it's necessarily safer than other medicines, or free from side effects. Do not take St John's wort with SSRI antidepressants, as there is evidence of adverse interaction. It may also decrease the effectiveness of oral contraceptives, some cholesterol-lowering medications and other commonly prescribed drugs. If you are taking a prescription medicine, check with your GP if it is safe to combine it with St John's wort.

Talking therapies

Traditional psychotherapy is based on retracing people's childhoods and early relationships to find out what makes them tick. Some people find it useful to unravel the reasons for their perceptions of life or to uncover patterns in personal relationships that mirror those with their parents, families and carers. It can be invaluable to become close to a caring, experienced person who will patiently work to uncover the past and journey towards the future. However, revisiting old traumas or hurts can keep someone caught in the past without noticing the present. Sometimes simply identifying what is wrong, and why, is not enough to make it right. Cognitive behaviour therapy is a combination of psychotherapy and behavioural therapy. Psychotherapy emphasises the importance of the personal meaning we place on things and how thinking patterns begin in childhood. Behavioural therapy pays close attention to the relationship between our problems, our behaviour and our thoughts.

The decision about which therapy to choose depends on the character and skills of the therapist and the personality of the person seeing them. The most important thing is to find a therapist whom you respect and trust.

Cognitive behavioural therapy (CBT)

CBT is based on a 'model' or theory that it's not events themselves that upset us, but the meanings we lend them. If our thoughts are too negative, it can block us seeing things or doing things that don't confirm what we believe is true. In other words, we continue to hold on to the same old thoughts and fail to learn anything new.

CBT describes a number of therapies that all have a similar approach to solving problems, which can range from sleeping difficulties or relationship problems, to drug and alcohol abuse or anxiety and depression. CBT works by changing people's attitudes and their behaviour. The therapies focus on the thoughts, images, beliefs and attitudes that we hold (our cognitive processes) and how this relates to the way we behave, as a way of dealing with emotional problems.

An important advantage of CBT is that it tends to be short. Sessions usually last about an hour and are once a week. Some treatments require as few as six to eight sessions. Between sessions you will be asked to put into practice what you have learned and may be given assignments. Client and therapist work together to understand what the problems are and to develop a new strategy for tackling them. CBT introduces you to a set of principles that you can apply whenever you need to, and which you can draw on if you experience a relapse.

One experience of cognitive behavioural theory

I was put on the SSRI, Seroxat, seven years ago and stayed on it for two. I only felt mildly better and still had depressive symptoms. I came off it after graduating from uni and moved to London to start a job. I started to experience a decline again after nine months to the point where I was off sick for a month and then left that job. My new GP put me on Cipramil and I recovered enough to hold down a new job and socialise, but I still had mild symptoms occasionally. I came off Cipramil after a year and had a relapse, so my GP advised me to go back on the medication. After another year, I stopped taking it again and my condition worsened.

At this point, I sought help privately from a psychiatrist and counsellor. My GP just wanted me to go back on Cipramil, but I wanted to look for a long-term solution as the drugs had never made me feel 100 per cent better anyway. The psychiatrist started me on a different type of drug called venlafaxine. I also had weekly sessions with my counsellor and learnt about cognitive behavioural therapy (CBT), which I found very positive. CBT helped me to understand the pattern of negative thoughts that I had fallen into over the years and made me realise that without working on them, my negative, and often incorrect, view of the world would only drag me back down. It's quite hard work to start with, but once you get used to CBT, it's a really useful coping mechanism.

My initial experiences of psychotherapy on the NHS hadn't been useful. I wanted someone to help me find answers and a way to feel better and cope better. All I got was lots of sympathy and tissue-handing, which was frankly even more depressing. I think there's a lot to be said for finding someone you can trust and talk to properly. The woman who finally helped me to get better was my third counsellor. I saw her for almost a year in the end and so we developed quite a bond, but I feel able to cope on my own now, though I am still on medication.

My psychiatrist checks me at regular intervals and at some point in the next few months I'm going to start coming off the drugs. That will be really scary, but the metaphor he used was that the medication was like restarting a clock that was running slow. Once the new batteries are in place (or the chemical levels in my brain) then you can take the 'crutch' of the drugs away and your body should compensate to keep the levels stable.

I hope he's right. Even if he is, I know that my depression is something that I will always be conscious of. But hopefully that very awareness, and the coping skills I have learnt over the years, will help to keep the really dark times from ever returning.

Goal setting

Another technique involves establishing goals for what you would like to achieve some time in the future.

Goal setting teaches you how to break down a journey into very small stages. This is very helpful if someone has become too depressed to deal with going out, or has lost the ability to cope with everyday tasks.

A friend or a counsellor can help plan every small step towards achieving the goal, making sure they are being supportive and that every step is realistic and achievable. Taking these steps lets someone who is frozen by depression slowly build on a series of successes.

This gradually changes the picture from one of despair, to one where new things can happen and be enjoyed.

An important part of this technique is to make sure every single step is just a tiny bit further along than the one before, and to never try to rush things along.

A weekly session may be necessary for six months or so to establish a pattern of achievement.

Depressed thinking can become a habit and it is useful to remember that it will take some time to learn another way of thinking to deal with stresses and challenges. It helps to meet regularly with the person who is helping you set goals for some time after the regular weekly sessions are completed, to help maintain the new approach until it also becomes a habit.

Physical therapy

Another theory holds that trauma and sadness get trapped in our bodies and that massage and guided exercise can help release these negative feelings. Reichian or bio-energy therapy offers a combination of focused deep massage and movement, with the therapist trained to carefully listen to the memories and feelings that may surface.

Dance therapy also uses movement to help people feel their bodies fully and express their emotions.

Creative therapy

There is an increasing move to use art and music to both express feelings and get in touch with the pleasure and satisfaction of creativity. When participants join a group they also learn to support others and to share their insights.

Horticulture and gardening

Another successful and popular way of moving forward is through joining a gardening or horticulture project. 'Green therapy' uses the combination of outside exercise, being in touch with the earth and working together to grow plants and vegetables. It can bring peace and fulfilment without focusing on depression or personal feelings at all.

Electro-convulsive therapy (ECT)

ECT involves sending an electric current through the brain to trigger a seizure, or fit, with the aim of relieving severe depression and some other conditions. The treatment is given under a general anaesthetic and using muscle relaxants, so that the muscles do not contract, and the body does not convulse during the fit.

ECT is usually regarded as a last resort, reserved for people who are suicidal or repeatedly self harming, or those experiencing severe depression who cannot tolerate drug therapies but require urgent treatment. It has been found very effective by some people for whom all other treatments have failed.

No-one seems to be able to give a clear explanation of how ECT works, and this is a cause of controversy. On the one hand, its critics describe it as crude and dangerous; on the other, its supporters defend it as an effective and life-saving technique.

Both critics and supporters have suggested that ECT works through causing brain damage. Some of the common adverse effects – drowsiness, confusion, forgetfulness, headaches, nausea – may subside quickly, but memory loss, apathy (emotional blunting), learning difficulties, and loss of creativity, drive and energy may last for weeks, months or even permanently.

For more information about ECT read the booklet *Making sense of ECT,* which is available on the Mind website www.mind.org.uk, or order it by writing to Mind Publications, 15-19 Broadway, London E15 4BQ or ringing 0844 448 4448.

Emergencies

When someone experiences a sudden crisis or the onset of severe depression, it is frightening both for them and for those around them.

Panic and anxiety attacks often accompany suicidal feelings. This can feel overwhelming and the person so affected may want to pace, talk rapidly or shout, or to curl up and withdraw as completely as possible.

What can you do?

Emergency visits from a GP or nurse, or a phone call to a mental health organisation, will reassure you that someone knows what is happening. This is the first step to getting out of the crisis situation.

It is vital to find someone to talk to and to regain a sense of calm. Some helplines are open 24 hours a day and the people answering are used to remaining calm and helpful through such situations. Often, unburdening yourself to a stranger is very useful, because they will not judge you and will keep everything you say confidential.

Talking, sharing the experience or even being able to be silent knowing someone is still there listening with you, really do help. A panic attack is temporary, but of course it is physically and emotionally painful and terrifying.

Sometimes it is worth accepting a hospital admission, to allow time for support to be put into place and for briefly letting professionals be responsible for your welfare. Hospitals nowadays do not keep people in for years – the aim is to help people back on their feet as soon as possible.

A very useful method is to 'feel' in your body where the suicidal urge is located. This seems to vary between the throat, chest, stomach and heart. Being aware of the physical sensation, consciously breathing more slowly and floating with it, reduces panic and helps you become calmer.

If you are with someone who is in a crisis

Phrases such as "calm down" or "stop panicking" often increase anxiety. Instead, use calm simple phrases such as "it will be ok" or "I am here, I'm not going". If they want it, hold or cuddle the person. They probably feel like a panicking child and need reassurance above all else.

If they have withdrawn and are huddled or rocking, stay with them quietly for a while, being there and providing the reassurance of your presence. If you need to go for help, tell them quietly what you are doing and when you will be back in the room.

It's a myth that those who talk about suicide do not act on their feelings. Take such thoughts seriously and let them know they are being listened to.

If you think medical help is needed, arrange it as quietly and matter-of-factly as possible. If someone has harmed themself or is behaving dangerously, do not comment on the behaviour. Say things like "I am going to get someone to help out" and if possible phone from another room. If you feel unsafe, say calmly "I am going into another room to get help. I will come back."

Showing that you understand and are not overwhelmed yourself is hugely reassuring. In crisis situations like bereavement, losing a partner, witnessing an accident or being suddenly made unemployed, you may think you can do nothing to help. Being there, clearly caring, is the most useful thing you can do.

Panic is contagious, so remember to breathe and relax. This will help both of you. It is often helpful to hold someone and gently tell them to breathe deeply, doing so yourself at the same time so that you become calmer in unison.

Remember to get support for yourself as well. Emergency helplines and medical or social services resources will be able to give you contacts. Use them or make sure you are talking to your friends and relatives and widening the support available – a network means a safety net in this situation and it's always good to have that.

Remember a crisis is a short-term emergency. This situation will change. You will not be expected to take decisions or offer this level of care forever. Be realistic about your own limits and get help from others.

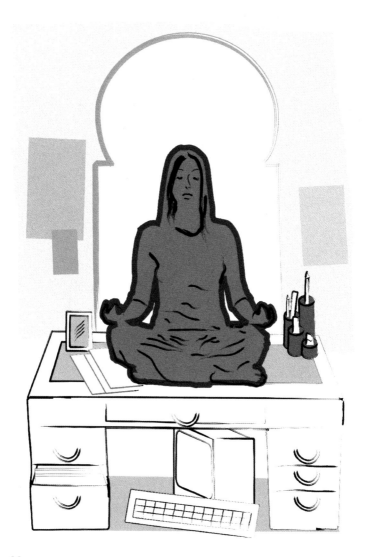

Work- and stress-related depression

Stress is usually seen as a negative thing, but originally the word just meant 'arousal' or 'stimulus'. When too much stress is not balanced by sensible strategies to address it, the stimulus turns into overload and can lead to a sense of helplessness and depression.

From birth we respond to stimuli by growing, learning and adapting. With praise and affirmation, a child learns how to overcome obstacles and sees change and challenges as exciting. If the environment we grow up in does not nurture us, it can be much harder to learn how to use stress to grow, and difficulties can feel overwhelming. Challenges are seen as obstacles when we have not learned the confidence to overcome them.

This can be changed by looking at your system of dealing with stress and learning to break down the causes. Each problem can be tackled with support and by looking at more manageable goals. Feelings of being overwhelmed and of hopelessness make this harder, so it is important to learn to relax and get allies to help you.

Learnt responses to stress

Some of the ways each person learns to deal with daily stress are appropriate in infancy or childhood, but can work against us as we get older. A method of avoiding or confronting stress that was just right in childhood can make everything worse in adulthood.

For example, think back to when you were five or six – how did you respond when your parents or teachers told you off, home life was difficult or a task seemed too hard for you? Some people learn to withdraw and become passive, others to be funny, cry or throw a temper tantrum, others seek to please even when frightened or angry.

Perhaps you learned to be very 'good' and pleasing when you were troubled. This may have worked to deflect a parent's anger when you were small, but may not be so appropriate or helpful for you when an employer or partner is being unreasonable in adult life. Withdrawing into silence may have saved you from a telling off when young, but may actively annoy people nowadays.

Denying responsibility and blaming someone else can be an understandable panic reaction, but will probably cause damage if it is your automatic response to criticism.

If you only have one habitual response to stress, you are likely to respond this way more and more as the situation gets worse. The problem that is causing the stress does not get addressed. You are likely to end up feeling helpless and depressed.

- How did you deal with difficult situations as a child?
- What is your usual method nowadays?
- Does it work well for you?
- What might be more effective?

When we are in danger, the two natural responses are 'fight or flight'. This can be translated as the desire to run away and ignore or avoid a situation, or to become angry and confrontational at the drop of a hat.

Neither of these responses is likely to be useful either in the workplace or social situations. It is necessary to step back, look at the cause of the stress and begin to take charge of your own response.

Firstly, it's important to acknowledge that a lot of situations are genuinely difficult. At work, at home or in a relationship, the combination of unwanted pressure and too little support can lead to deep anxiety and a reduction in the ability to cope. This does not mean you're at fault. There are established procedures to address problems at work.

Studies into employment practices have shown the following causes of poor performance and consequent stress at work:

- having a job that is too difficult or too easy for you,

or one that does not match your skills, experience and expectations

- repetitive tasks over which you have no control
- deadline pressures
- poor working conditions, including noise, poor lighting and lack of safety precautions
- lack of clarity about your role and responsibilities
- lack of management support
- bullying
- exclusion from the mainstream workforce owing to factors such as race or gender
- inadequate procedures to challenge discrimination
- lack of opportunities for career development or promotion
- organisational changes in which you have no say.

Symptoms of stress in these situations include:

- resentment
- sleeplessness
- inability to concentrate
- boredom and apathy
- irritability
- anxiety and depression.

Stepping back and breaking the problem down, then getting support to deal with it can help.

Changing the work environment

Build your support network. Share ideas, good practices and skills with co-workers.

Discuss your workload with a supervisor or manager and clarify your areas of expertise, targets and workload.

Join an assertiveness class. This can build your ability to politely negotiate compromises if you are experiencing unreasonable demands.

Limit long hours. Keep a time-sheet if necessary, to show that you are working hard but the contracted hours are not sufficient for the tasks required of you.

Seek careers advice to find ways of shifting your skills and experience into more satisfying work. There are many home study, part-time and evening courses available at all levels to provide training, many free or with bursaries available. learndirect gives free, impartial advice. You can find the details under *Useful organisations* on page 117.

Look after yourself with attention to healthy eating. Take a walk in your lunch break, try to have a three-minute stretch and deep breathing session rather than a cigarette, get to bed on time regularly and learn a relaxation technique.

Know your rights

1   Be aware of your company's policies on bullying, discrimination and access to support.   ▶

2   Contact the Citizens Advice Bureau (CAB) or your union official to check if you can get support to improve health and safety or interpersonal issues at work.

3   Contact Employment Tribunals or Acas, the publicly funded organisation responsible for improving employment relations, for advice on pursuing a complaint against your employer.

4   Taking time off owing to emotional distress or mental ill health is as valid as any other type of sick leave. If you need to do this, ensure you have a note from your GP and ask for union or CAB help to ensure your employer supports your re-entry into work.

Outside the workplace

Try to find ways to relax – turning to alcohol or comfort eating will not help in the long term. Have you tried simple physical relaxation techniques? A full relaxation session is described in chapter four, therapeutic massage and swimming are also excellent. No job is important enough to let it damage your health. If it is making you ill, then start by listing the reasons you are still there.

If you mostly like your job, what needs to be changed? Decide who, within or outside the organisation, could help with this. Perhaps, after all, it's time to move on, but bear in mind that a time of high stress might not be the best time to make a dramatic decision.

What would you rather be doing?

What is the first step to getting there?

List your skills and experience. See the next three months as the route to taking that first step. Get a training prospectus, talk to friends, your partner, your supervisor or a counsellor about your plans.

If possible, save hard to have enough money for a break. And remember that life is all about change and this is not a permanent situation.

Being tense and stressed out is very tiring, and exhaustion can be both a symptom and a cause of depression. As well as looking at the problems at work and getting help to deal with them, look after yourself physically.

Redundancy and unemployment

Working patterns have changed dramatically in the past decade. People, who have grown up expecting to remain in a job for life and then retire with a pension, are faced with shorter-term periods of work and the frightening possibility of financial uncertainty – the result can be stress, anxiety and depression.

There are no easy solutions, but there are several initiatives being developed in response to this national problem.

- learndirect and other training and education programmes aim to give people support and information to retrain and gain employable skills to start a new career path.

- Legislation is making it illegal to discriminate against job applicants on the grounds of age.

- There are advisors at Jobcentres, offering practical support to gain work placements and qualifications and to write CVs and applications.

- If your redundancy seems unfair or focused on the post-holder rather than the post, contact Acas immediately on being informed and take advice on appeals.

There is no shame in being made redundant. People at all levels in a wide range of organisations may have to go through this experience. Skills and experience are transferable. After the shock of realising a job has been cut or a firm is shutting down, it is worth listing all the skills gained during that period of work. Many are applicable to other forms of work, for example, supervision and management skills can be taken from industry into service or public settings. Use of practical skills shows that a person has the ability to learn and put into practice complicated manual training.

This is a time to take a step back and assess what you really want. There are advisors and experts to guide you into areas of work where new recruits are needed.

Friends and partners of someone who has been made redundant or who is unemployed need to remember how much self-esteem is attached to work.

Uncharacteristic irritation or short temper can be symptoms of panic and depression. Even relatively short periods of unemployment can make people feel helpless and angry. Try to stand back and not respond with anger.

During this stressful time it is a good idea to take advantage of the calm, objective professional help available for advice and support.

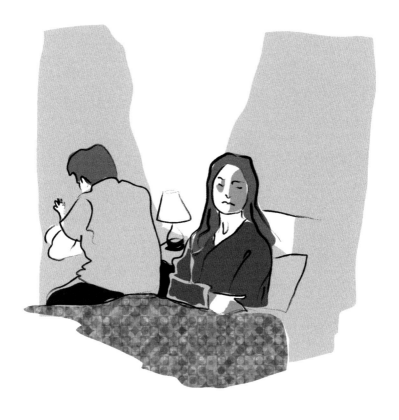

Post-natal depression

Post-natal depression (PND) affects two out of ten mothers in the months after giving birth. It is not the 'baby blues' – a short period of weepiness that occurs for many women three or four days after having the baby and lifts naturally within a week or so. Post-natal depression usually begins after this. It is longer lasting and can affect the woman's relationship with the baby and all the people around her.

PND is such a common condition that many doctors and health visitors are trained to identify it as part of post-natal care. Unfortunately, not all GP practices are trained to do this and of course not everyone has a good relationship with their doctor. There is still help available if this is true for you, so please read on.

Although it lifts eventually, untreated PND can last for weeks, months or even a couple of years. When identified and treated early it will steadily improve and not return.

Symptoms of PND

Feeling unhappy, weepy and low most of the time – the feelings can be worse at particular times of the day, most usually the morning and late afternoon. Lack of interest in or dislike of the baby can be symptoms and this is made worse by guilt and feelings of failure. Enjoyment disappears.

Tiredness All new parents are tired, but a woman experiencing PND feels completely exhausted to the point where she may think she is severely physically ill. This is often accompanied by an inability to relax or sleep, even when someone else is taking care of the baby to give her a break.

Irritability This can become a daily feeling, causing the mother to snap at older children, or be constantly on edge with the baby and be unable to endure the baby's crying. Irritability is often shown most of all to partners and family, who may wonder why they 'always seem in the wrong'. This sometimes causes them to snap back, withdraw or get depressed themselves.

Changes in eating patterns Like other forms of depression, PND can lead either to a loss of appetite and disgust with food, or to overeating. Not eating makes the mother even less able to find the energy to undertake her own or the baby's care. Overeating can affect her self-image and slow the usual regaining of a comfortable post-natal body weight.

Panic attacks and acute anxiety about the day-to-day care of the baby can overwhelm even the most capable mothers. Feelings of hostility or fear of the baby can lead to fantasies of abandoning or even harming the child. Mothers may experience an exaggerated fear that the baby has stopped breathing, is ill or at risk of cot death. This can make mothers scared to be alone with their babies and may cause them to become clingy and desperate with their partner or friends.

Not coping The combination of exhaustion, panic and feelings of detachment, creates feelings of helplessness. Establishing a routine or being able to start everyday tasks seem difficult or impossible.

Although PND is very common, it is a serious, frightening and overwhelming condition. Women experiencing it need practical, emotional and medical support as early as possible.

Most women will recover spontaneously, but this can take many months. During this time, the important early relationship with the baby will be affected, so it benefits everyone if help is sought as soon as possible.

Causes

As with all types of depression, there is a variety of expert opinions on the causes of PND. There may well be links between the different causes, so they are known collectively as 'risk factors'.

These can be summarised as follows:

1 Many women react strongly to the hormonal changes that take place after giving birth. Some women begin to feel depressed during pregnancy, again possibly because of a reaction to hormonal changes, others will feel increasingly low in the weeks afterwards.

2 There are links between women who experience pre-menstrual tension and those who also suffer PND.

3 Women who have suffered depression in their teens and 20s or have had PND with previous babies are particularly susceptible.

4 Lone parenting or lack of support from a partner can create loneliness and exhaustion leading to depression.

5 Loss of a parent during the mother's own childhood.

6 Premature birth of the baby.

7 Unexpected disability or illness in the newborn.

8 A disappointing or very difficult birth experience.

9 Practical difficulties with housing, income or redundancy during pregnancy.

10 Emotional overload including bereavement, partnership breakdown or poor relationships with the extended family.

11 Moving away from familiar surroundings during pregnancy or early parenthood.

Although some women are vulnerable to PND even when these factors are not present, the more risk factors a woman has, the more likely she is to become depressed at this time. Health visitors, who visit all families in the weeks after giving birth, are trained to recognise the symptoms and put you in touch with support networks. There is also a network of family support organisations.

What can be done to help?

If your depression lasts longer than a few days you should discuss it with your health visitor. They may have a short questionnaire called the Edinburgh Scale, which they will use to ask you about your feelings.

You do not have to go on suffering in the hope that it will go away. PND is a very real condition. Great care needs to be taken with drugs during pregnancy and after giving birth. A balance has to be struck between the needs of the mother-to-be and the possible risk to the unborn child, particularly in the first three months of pregnancy. After the birth, a nursing mother is likely to pass any drugs she is taking to her baby through her breast milk. Antidepressants are powerful drugs, and very little is known about their effect on unborn children or babies being breast fed. Tricyclic antidepressants given in late pregnancy have been associated with withdrawal symptoms in newborn babies. Every alternative to drugs should be explored. With help and support, drugs may be unnecessary.

If you feel like screaming, put the baby safely in its bed then go into the bathroom, shut the door and shout or cry if you want to. You do not have to live up to an unrealistically rosy view of motherhood. Everyone finds it difficult sometimes.

Be good to yourself. Make the best of the good times, however rare they are now. They will probably become more frequent as you move on from this stage – and there is practical social and emotional support available for you and your baby. The feelings are not your fault and you will move on from this. As you recover, the bad days get fewer and further apart and the good days increase.

It is important to eat well, take up all offers of a break and to get out and not stay trapped in the home all day. If these things also feel too much for you, please talk to your health visitor, GP or local family support project as soon as you can, because there is help available.

When you see the doctor it may help to take along your partner, a relative or friend. Your midwife, health visitor or community nurse can also give you help and support. She can put you in touch with groups that offer support or have a network of other mothers who have successfully recovered from PND. They know what you are going through and how to help.

How can partners and friends help?

You may find yourself becoming agitated or depressed as well. It can be very wearing to live with a new baby *and* someone suffering PND. Many fathers become depressed, too, after the birth of a baby, so you should not feel guilty.

> You may be angry about your partner's depression or feel distressed and helpless.
>
> You may need to encourage her to seek help or to go together.
>
> Above all, be patient and remember the condition is temporary.

Practical and emotional help you can give:

- Mothers with PND are often exceptionally sensitive to what is said to them. Practical support is easier to interpret as helpful than advice.

- Shopping, cooking and tidying up are all hugely helpful. Mothering is a full-time task in the early weeks.

- Mothers should be allowed to express their fluctuating emotions. It is unhelpful to be told to pull yourself together.

- Recovery is not easy and will not always happen quickly, but it will come.

- Sometimes it is easier to talk outside our immediate circle of friends and family. This is not a reflection on those close to the mother. It can be a big step to seek outside help, but if she feels embarrassed or ashamed of her feelings, it is much better that they are expressed rather than bottled up.

- Post-natal depression brings real suffering and getting help early can save the family from months of this unpleasant condition.

Talking it through: counselling and therapy

Studies have shown that as little as an hour a week of talking to a trained health visitor can significantly reduce post-natal depression. Some mothers need this time on their own, others want to include a partner to move forward together. You don't necessarily need to find out what caused the PND. It is still helpful to talk over the pain or anxiety you are experiencing with a nonjudgemental listener.

Groups

In many areas, there are self-help groups of women who have had similar experiences. It can be a relief to find you are not alone. Your health visitor may even run such a group. Self-help groups allow you to honestly express your feelings in a setting where others understand.

Relating to your baby

When someone is deeply depressed, it is difficult or impossible to feel loving and attentive towards the baby. Sometimes mothers cannot feel any pleasure in the baby. Sometimes they feel fiercely protective to the point that they become intensely anxious most of the time.

If there is a local baby massage group, join it. This has been shown to help with PND. It creates a safe, comfortable place for you to get to touch and attend to the baby with other mothers around you.

Get as much rest as possible. Cat naps, baths, a sit down in the sun in the park, will all give you much needed time for yourself. Make sure you get out every day. Exercise helps you relax and being out will give you a break from being alone with the baby's demands.

Remember it is completely unnatural for a woman to be alone all day with a small baby. That is why so many mother and baby groups exist – to create the informal networks our grandmothers took for granted. There will always be other mothers there who don't know anyone yet. Your baby will give you an excellent excuse not to chat if you don't feel like it, and you can always have a look and see who is around for when you do.

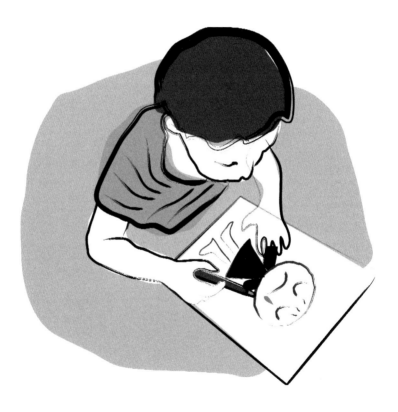

Depression among younger people

Children as young as two or three can become deeply depressed. The signals can include regression to babyish behaviour, bedwetting, rage, apathy, anxiety and clinginess. This can start after illness, when there has been a family trauma such as a bereavement or marital breakdown, after a house move or when a new brother or sister arrives.

Parents may be involved in their own feelings to the extent that they cannot respond to the child. If a baby does not get the attention they are calling for, either through crying or demanding, she will finally give up asking. This can then turn into childhood depression, where the little one does not learn how to get their needs met and stops trying.

If this happens it can be helped by asking the health visitor or local Sure Start, Home Start or Family Support Project to step in. By being supported to play together, respond to the child and listen to them, the parent comes back into focus and the child is helped to relearn how to ask for the nurturing they need.

With a young child, there is day care and support group help available through the health visitor. The health visitor sees hundreds of families and will not judge you for asking.

School age children will have a familiar teacher they see every day. Tell them if there has been something upsetting for your child, asking for it to remain in confidence. If the child is upset about school, it's worth talking to the head teacher and asking for a lunchtime helper or classroom assistant to offer extra care for a while.

Ask for help if you cannot manage alone. Parenting is a complicated, highly emotional business and everyone needs help and advice sometimes. Remember too that however young a child is they will be emotionally affected by family upsets. They are not trying to further upset you with their behaviour, but trying to let you know they want some help too. Let your child's teacher know why their behaviour may have changed, for example, if you are going through a divorce or separation from your partner.

Young children need contact and cuddles as much as they need intellectual and social stimulation. Try to put aside a time each day for a story on your lap or to remember to sit with your arm round them while watching TV.

Reassurance, praise, a regular routine and positive attention from their carers build up a child's confidence remarkably quickly after a period of upset.

Teenage depression

Below are the examples of two teenagers who have recently experienced depression.

James, aged 16

James has felt depressed on and off since he was about nine. After a short period of being badly bullied on starting secondary school, the feelings became worse. He has learnt some ways of coping with the feelings, particularly by doing martial arts to release his anger, and by talking to two friends who sometimes feel the same way.

Now, at 16, the depression has lessened significantly. Having learned to recognise the feelings, he draws and writes when they start, which also helps. This is his advice:

When I'm depressed I feel really out of body, lethargic and permanently exhausted. I am cynical about everything and don't care about my friends. I feel depressed thinking about school, going there, being there. I don't like my school personality but don't seem to be able to switch into my home one when I'm there.

Teenage depression affects a lot of people, but if you are suffering from depression as a teenager you will probably be feeling isolated and unique. Fluctuating hormones, which are difficult to predict and deal with, cause some teenage depression. A regular sleep pattern and regular meals and snacks can help to deal with this form of depression. Low blood sugar can cause depression by itself or also aggravate existing depression.

People with depression may feel a wide range of emotions, paranoia, fear, anger or just sadness. It is far more effective to talk to someone else if you are feeling depressed rather than trying to deal with your depression on your own. You may want to talk to a doctor or school counsellor, or if you are nervous or unsure about talking to them then just talk to a family member. A close friend can be useful to talk to; you may well discover that what you are feeling is not unusual.

It is highly important to find an outlet for any emotions connected to depression. Drawing, writing and physical exercise, even just going for a short walk, can all help lift depression temporarily. If you are feeling depressed, get as much sleep as you can. Exhaustion can intensify many of the emotions or feelings associated with depression, such as sadness, lethargy or paranoia. Learning to acknowledge your own periods of depression when they happen can be helpful in finding a short- or longer-term way out.

Anna, aged 13

I get really weepy for no reason and then just want to hide away and not see anyone. Twice I have been crying too much to go to school in the morning. This happens before my period. I worry about my exams. My mum wants me to do homework every day and I feel tired all the time and want to sleep or chill out and then I get really sad and despairing. When I cry, my parents let me curl up and stay at home and that helps, but there is still all the work to catch up on afterwards.

It is easy to dismiss teenage depression as 'just hormones'. However, the incidence of suicide and attempted suicide in young people is rising and increased services to help them are being set up in response. YoungMinds, Connexions and Samaritans have trained workers to listen to and support young people and their parents.

Symptoms of depression are not always weepiness or lethargy – rage and panic, avoiding homework, inattention in class or repeated stomach- and headaches may be signs, too.

Living with teenagers

This can be deeply stressful. Parents have lost the caring role with younger children, which can give a lot of satisfaction, and find themselves living with teenagers who challenge and argue, often seeming to really dislike and resent the adults around them.

Don't take it personally. If teenagers didn't become independent, they would not be able to grow up.

It is important to remember that the closer you are to a child, the more difficult it will be for you to separate. They will, of course, continue to develop on their own and sound foundations of love and trust will remain.

Keep boundaries. Act with warmth but firmly, even if this is not how you feel. The young person will feel safer even if they continue to rebel. Imagine how you would like to be talked to if roles were reversed. Telling someone to do something is always more effective if you can explain rather than dictate or rant. When you want to shout back, remember this is quite normal, you are not a monster. You are the adult and if you can stay calm, or even remove yourself from the room, it is more effective than getting drawn into battles.

Go out and reclaim your own adult life. It hurts when the child you love has temporarily changed into a sullen or aggressive housemate. You deserve to have a good time yourself, so actively seek out a class, increase your social life or find ways of treating yourself.

Join a parents' group and allow yourself to express your feelings with others going through the same thing. Not only will you realise that you aren't alone in the situation, you may even have a laugh sometimes. Remember this is usually a temporary phase.

What helps?

All children and teenagers have to experience stressful situations, and learn to cope with them, as part of growing up.

It is very important to acknowledge to them that they are going through a difficult time and that it is a positive stage leading on to something else.

Suggest small steps to tackle a problem.

- Get support for yourself if the teenager is being angry and aggressive with you. Getting into battles that you both desperately want to win can send tension spiralling out of control. Try to step back and ask "is this really so important?" Let them have the last word sometimes, while being firm about who the adult is and what is unacceptable to you.

- Show them they have your support in a difficult situation.

- Listen to them and ask how you can help. Try to offer rewards rather than punishments to help establish a routine. For example, can you make a favourite snack for them to eat before homework? Would they swap a permitted allowance of TV or computer time in exchange for an agreed amount of study?

- Laughing them out of it or teasing about moodiness can feel like the final blow to a child who is 'acting out' to show their distress.

- Try to establish firm, kind boundaries, keeping in mind the need to help them feel secure.

- Do you know if anything is wrong at school or with their friends?

- Bullying can destroy a child's self-esteem. If this is happening to your child, take their side. Schools have established codes to tackle the problem. Approach a class teacher in confidence and talk over what's happening and ensure that your child gets help.

- If the child is distressed by behaviour that seems minor to you, please try to consider what they are feeling and take it seriously. Being told off or advised to stand up for themselves will make them feel more isolated.

- If they are repeatedly ill with no apparent cause – go to the doctor together. It might be helpful to talk to the GP alone first to let them know your child needs reassurance and should be encouraged to talk over any hidden worries.

- Fluctuating hormones, changing body shape, feelings of alienation or inadequacy are all part of adolescence. Acknowledge this and reassure them that they are not alone. Don't tease them about an area of self-consciousness.

- Try to find something they are proud of about themselves and encourage it.

- Make sure their time is not completely taken over by schoolwork. Leisure time, chilling out and doing nothing are very important as well.

- Can you find a weekend activity with no pressure to achieve attached to it?

The child's body is growing, they are learning about their place in the world and taking in some of the realities about the human condition even the wisest adult finds difficult to accept. Listen to them as much as you can.

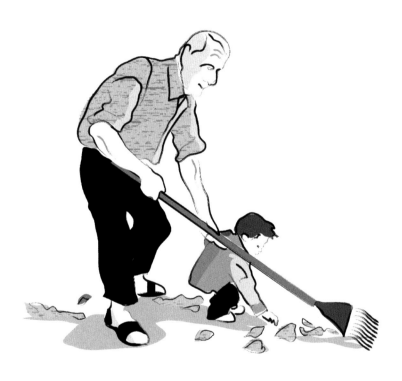

Growing older and coping with loss

"You're having a mid-life crisis!"

This annoying little phrase is used to explain anything from mild discontent, through to someone completely re-examining all their life's choices and values, at any time between the ages of 35 and 60.

Although throw-away explanations like this are little help, 'crisis' is a good term for describing some of the deep-seated feelings of anxiety and panic which may be experienced.

Realisations made about life choices in your late 30s and early 40s can be frightening and depressing:

• Children are growing up and staging the dramas of their teenage years.

• Menopause confronts women with the loss of their youth and fertility.

• Many men experience a huge shift in self-image, to which it can be difficult to adjust.

• Men and women may realise they do not enjoy their chosen career or family life.

- We may be confronted with the death of parents and friends, and with the reality of our own mortality.

Naturally, such feelings can trigger a time of reappraisal and transition.

Society places huge emphasis on youth, but middle age can also be a time of great growth and deep contentment. Understanding what we want to be and do, allows us to be far less dependent on other people's approval. Self-knowledge, increased self-confidence and the wisdom of experience make the journey into the second half of our lives a fascinating experience, but there are, of course, obstacles on the way.

Menopause

Many women think it is inevitable that the menopause will bring depression – some even expect to be miserable as they get older. In fact, many women feel happier, less moody and increasingly fulfilled as they move through their 40s and 50s.

Women seem more likely than men to experience depression sometime during their lives. This has led to research into possible links between depression and fluctuations in hormone levels. Mood changes can affect some women in similar ways when they experience menstruation, post-natal depression and the period directly before menopause, which is called the peri-menopause.

Other symptoms of menopause are similar to those of depression, like sleeplessness, irritability, extreme tiredness and mood swings. Some of the physical symptoms are worrying or distressing, especially heavy bleeding or flooding, and hot flushes and sweats. Taking the hormone progesterone often controls these symptoms, but it can have side effects such as weight gain and depression.

A lot more research is needed in this area; however, links between the body's decreased production of the 'happy' hormone, oestrogen, and depression seem to be experienced by many women. It is worth getting medical advice about whether a hormone supplement might help you, or to go to an alternative practitioner to think about the many natural herbs and foods that can help in this time.

The peri-menopause is associated with the gradual decrease in production of oestrogen. However, depression may also be caused by other changes in your life, low thyroid production, tiredness due to overwork or any number of other factors. It makes sense, therefore, to have a full health check rather than to just assume your feelings are due to your age or to menopause.

Practical sources of help

Eating a well balanced diet is important, as is increasing your intake of iron and vitamin B6, which will help with tiredness due to excessive bleeding and balance the body's reaction to reducing oestrogen levels. Try to reduce caffeine, sugar and chocolate intake over a few weeks and see if that affects your mood.

Many people need less sleep as they get older, however, long sleepless anxious nights are a common sign of depression and anxiety. As so often with depression, it is probably time to think about looking after yourself now. Do you have a bedtime routine? Set one by having a warm bath half an hour before bed. Keep caffeine- or chocolate-based drinks for earlier in the day and choose something soothing and milky for the evening. Or try camomile tea, which has been used around the world for centuries.

Stress makes depression worse. What worries you at the moment? It is worth trying a simple relaxation technique, lying down or sitting in a comfortable chair during the evening and concentrating on telling yourself it is evening, your thoughts are something you can control. Let your worries go, decide instead to think about your breathing. Let your shoulders sink down and relax with each long outward breath, spend ten minutes letting your face, your neck and your shoulders relax in response to your own deep, even breathing (see chapter four).

Spend time with other people. If you live alone or are by yourself a lot, try to go out every day. Consider going to the library to research places you can meet people, or to find details of a class or support group. Sometimes nurses in a GP or Wellwoman surgery can set up menopause groups for women to meet, share what works for them and learn what is going on physically for them. Would that be useful for you? Check it out.

Exercise is a good way of moving on through the physical discomfort of early menopausal symptoms. Walking slightly faster than usual, swimming a couple of times a week, getting off the bus or train a stop early or joining a beginners' exercise class will all help. Even ten minutes extra exercise a day makes a significant difference in a short time.

Depression makes it difficult to enjoy everyday activities. If you can dip into doing pleasurable things even if you don't feel like it, sooner or later some things will feel enjoyable again. It is really worth persevering so that the structure is there to feel good again when you are ready.

You will get through this time and feel better again. Many women have spent much of their lives looking after others and they have the skills to look after themselves too. What can you start with?

There is practical, medical and social support out there for you. You have taken an important step by beginning to look at ways of getting help. Fortunately, depression is a treatable condition and there are many options available for supporting you through menopause.

Remember – post-menopausal women experience significantly less depression than other groups in society. Depression is definitely not a consequence of ageing for most women and it does not have to be for you.

Caring for older parents

It is not unusual for people in middle life to have joint caring roles, looking after their own children while finding themselves living with and caring for elderly relatives.

Get support for yourself, too, if this is your situation.

Bring in help with practical tasks and ensure no one becomes the sole carer by default. If there are two parents or older children in a household, a simple rota for tasks such as vacuum cleaning or washing up makes the caring role a shared part of family life, not a burden.

Take time away and don't become completely focused on the home. There is a network of carers' organisations that may be able to offer practical and social support and information, as well as advice on respite care, lunch clubs and health issues.

Don't feel guilty – don't feel you have to do everything yourself. People live to a great age nowadays and services are being developed to respond to this. It is just as enjoyable for an older person to have time out and about socialising as it is for carers to spend time in another role.

Separation and divorce

This is one of the most traumatic experiences people go through and can leave them feeling very lonely and unsupported. Yet nearly half of marriages end in separation. Many people find that middle age brings about a desire to move away from a long relationship. Maybe one partner wishes to remain together while the other does not. Of course, for someone who is unwillingly separated that means having to redefine who they are and how to reshape the next part of their lives. This can be terrible shock and takes time to come to terms with.

Giving support

If you are trying to support someone through this period, it is helpful to remember not to criticise the person who has left. Acknowledge the sadness or anger – which it is normal to feel – by saying something open like "you must feel really sad", rather than "you're better off without them". Who would like to think they had been married to someone other people did not actually like or respect?

Allow time for the grieving process. For several weeks or months, it can be helpful to just drop round and be friendly and caring rather than hoping the person will join in socialising or quickly start looking for a new partner. Offer your company for simple, undemanding social activities like going to the cinema or shopping.

But remember not to be insistent; the person may not be ready to face social situations.

Not working

Redundancy and unemployment can be factors in depression at any stage of life (see chapter six). They often appear more desperate and devoid of positive outcomes for people in middle or later life, as the job market can seem oriented around younger people.

Retirement may have an impact on your relationships and it can be harder to cope with spending 24 hours a day with your partner than either of you imagined. You may feel anxious about the future, and worried about maintaining your standard of living.

Depending on the individual, life during retirement may be more or less similar to earlier life in terms of occupations, interests and aims. However, most people find that they have far more free time during retirement, even if they had not been previously occupied by full-time employment. This increase in leisure time can be used to pursue the opportunities on offer for continued social, intellectual and spiritual development.

Whatever you choose to do, most older people, no less than younger adults, find that it is important to keep or develop interests, stay – or become more – active and develop a regular structure to their day.

Depression in later life

Depression affects older people more than any other demographic group. This is because older people face more events and situations that may trigger depression: physical illness and debilitating physical conditions, bereavement, poverty and isolation.

As an older person experiencing depression, you may find that your symptoms are mistaken for other ailments. This is because symptoms can often differ from those experienced in younger age groups. Symptoms of depression such as agitation and anxiety, can be confused in later years with Parkinson's or Alzheimer's disease. They may also be confused with thyroid disorders, strokes or heart disease, or as a side effect of medication (which they can sometimes be). However, if you have depression it can prevent or delay recovery from other illnesses and injuries.

Older people who have depression, or other forms of mental distress, are sometimes misdiagnosed as having dementia, but depression is more common. The symptoms that can be misdiagnosed include forgetfulness, lack of concentration and loss of thinking ability. In fact, someone with depression is likely to be aware of these problems and be able to discuss them, while someone with dementia is not.

If you think you may have depression which has been misdiagnosed, discuss these concerns with your GP and, if necessary, get a second opinion. It is also your right to ask for a comprehensive assessment, which would involve specialists in psychiatry and neurology.

Although depression can appear for the first time in later years, it can also strike anyone at any stage of life. If you are an older person who has had recurrent or chronic depression since earlier life, you may be familiar with its causes and alert to your symptoms. You may have learnt the best ways to manage or recover from your condition over many years. However, there may also be other ways to alleviate depression that you might find helpful.

You may experience interactions between antidepressants and medication you are taking for physical conditions. It is also worth being aware that some medications can actually cause depression as a side effect.

Talking about your feelings, fears and negative thoughts, as well as how to manage them, can help to alleviate depression.

Living with loss – grief, mourning and recovery

In Western society, the grieving process is often a lonely one. Everyone will inevitably lose people close to them, but we no longer experience the death of family, friends, neighbours and acquaintances as part of an extended community's everyday life.

Although we witness wholesale death on the TV and in newspapers every day, the central rituals of mourning are absent from most people's lives until the passing of someone close brings death home. This means that someone who has lost a close friend or relative may feel very alone, without companions who understand how to help and be around.

Sadness is a normal part of mourning. The numbing effect of grief can be a buffer to protect someone from the immediate shock of loss. In the weeks and months after bereavement most people slowly come to terms with their loss, but sometimes they can become trapped in grief and need ongoing help in order to move on.

How to help someone undergoing bereavement

Acknowledge a person's grief. It is very tempting to try to distract someone from their mourning, especially if their way of expressing it makes their companions feel frightened, sad or angry themselves. Yet having someone around who is attentive, or simply 'there', is hugely helpful.

Let the person cry. In many societies, people are actively encouraged to weep and howl when they are bereaved. Rituals of communal crying and protest against death, allow the immediate family to be accompanied and recognised in their feelings. In Britain, such displays of feeling are unusual and often frowned upon. But if the natural urge to cry and rage is suppressed, where does it go? Depression means 'pushed down' and in this situation it is far healthier to allow someone to express their emotions. If you are uncomfortable with this, it might be better to acknowledge your discomfort and offer practical, rather than emotional, support.

One mother's experience

When I lost my baby, my neighbour came round. I was crying and sobbing all over the place, Anna was not even dressed or her nappy changed, the place was in chaos. Sally, my neighbour, took a look round and she said "I can't cope with the feelings but I could come round for a bit and look after Anna and do your washing and things like that". It really made a difference, she came round for six or seven weeks and kept the place together for me and I didn't have to talk but I knew she was there.

Let the bereaved person repeat themself – revisiting the fact of the death is an important part of grieving. Some theories explain this by saying that only by going over the memory of the person dying can we accept it has really happened. Trying to distract someone or help them move on before they are ready may stop their natural healing.

It might be useful to have an informal rota of people that can keep visiting or telephoning, so that no one person bears the whole brunt of someone's grief. There are also several support groups available, including organisations offering home-visiting volunteers who have gone through similar experiences themselves and have taken training to support others.

Traditionally, communities would take meals round to those affected by death and share practical tasks among themselves, ensuring the bereaved were kept warm, fed and that funeral arrangements taken care of.

Do not try to hurry someone through the stages of mourning. Try to remain aware that each person needs to revisit every stage several times and that eccentric or angry behaviour is part of this. It does not mean a visitor is doing something wrong. Arguing or trying to rationalise their emotions may be unhelpful.

If you are very worried that someone may be at risk of suicide or harming themselves (see the section on *Emergencies,* page 62), try and talk calmly with them about it. Perhaps they just need to express such impulses and will be reassured that someone is there to listen. Talking to someone from Cruse Bereavement Care, Samaritans or Mind*info*Line, can let them know they are not alone and that other people understand and care.

In the longer term, a bereaved person may find that most of their support has disappeared and people seem to expect them to have moved on. This can be a very lonely time. Missing someone is a way of keeping them alive and in our thoughts. Birthdays, anniversaries, Christmas and holidays are all painful reminders. It can be a comfort to phone or visit at such times, to talk through memories and look at photos, so the dead person is remembered with affection and love.

Talking about someone who has died does not have to be painful. Shared memories can bring real warmth and recognition, especially if people tend to shy away from mentioning the dead person's name. If a long-term partner or a beloved child has died, they are still part of the family and it is good to be able to know they are still important and acknowledged.

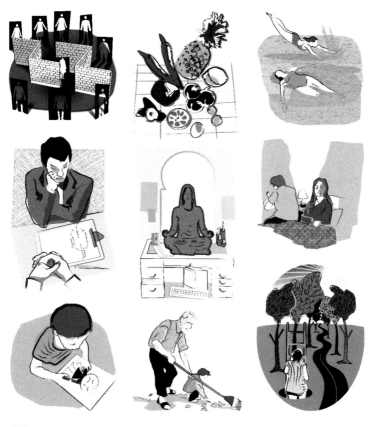

The sun also rises

A large percentage of people experience depression at some time during their lives. Learning strategies for coping is an essential part of reconnecting with mainstream life. If you can teach yourself to acknowledge when and how each bout of depression starts, you are on your way to managing the feelings, getting help in the situations which trigger them and short-circuiting the cycle.

Nobody seeks depression. Depression is not a conscious choice and no one is to blame. Yet, you can make a choice to act and think differently and slowly move into another approach to your life. Even if the physical and emotional symptoms continue, seeking and using help will provide tools to rebuild coping techniques and gain comfort.

Because depression feeds off itself, outside support is usually invaluable – isolation makes things worse. This help can be social, medical, from a formal set-up or from friends and family. Usually people experiencing severe depression need to use several methods to move forwards and it can take a lot of time and patience.

If friends, family or partners are unable to cope, they can also get information, advice and support from the network of agencies available. This is a healthy and sensible response, because using the available pool of expertise makes it easier to offer useful and sustainable support without becoming overwhelmed.

Some themes have recurred throughout this book:

- Get help when you feel depressed – it's there and some of it will be appropriate and useful for you.

- Don't feel guilty about your feelings. They are common across all sectors of society and are part of being a responsive, sensitive person.

- Anger and sadness are normal responses to loss, stress, fear and isolation. Facing the reasons you feel like this will allow you to cope with situations, as well as with your feelings.

- Using small steps to recovery gives you back control over your feelings and helps you build new habitual responses, which will be useful next time something stressful occurs.

- You do not have to battle this alone.

Please read through the list of self-help groups and agencies at the end of the book. It would be worth searching on the web, emailing or ringing for information or contacts now, so they are available when you need them.

Every person experiences depression individually, so everyone needs a personal, tailor-made package of support and help. If one way does not suit you, try another – with a range from self-help groups and lifestyle adjustments, through to modern pharmaceutical and talking therapies, shopping around and taking advice will allow you to find what suits you best.

Above all, know you can be helped. Accept help and company on this journey and remember you are not alone. There is joy, pleasure, kindness and comfort out there too. You can learn how to rediscover these and let them back into your life.

Moving on from depression

Useful organisations

General

Carers UK

20-25 Glasshouse Yard, London EC1A 4JT,
helpline: 0808 808 7777, tel: 020 7490 8818,
fax: 020 7490 8824, email: info@carersuk.org,
website: www.carersuk.org
Information and advice on all aspects of caring.

Cruse Bereavement Care

Cruse House, 126 Sheen Road, Richmond TW9 1UR,
helpline: 0870 167 1677,
young person's helpline: 0808 808 1677,
helpline email: helpline@crusebereavementcare.org.uk,
tel: 020 8939 9530, fax: 020 8940 7638,
email: info@crusebereavementcare.org.uk,
website: www.crusebereavementcare.org.uk

Depression Alliance

212 Spitfire Studios, 63-71 Collier Street, London N1 9BE,
tel: 0845 123 2320,
email: information@depressionalliance.org,
website: www.depressionalliance.org
Provides information and support.

Eating Disorders Association
103 Prince of Wales Road, Norwich NR1 1DW,
helpline: 0845 634 1414, helpline email:
helpmail@edauk.com, tel: 0870 770 3256,
textphone: 01603 753 322, fax: 01603 664 915,
email: info@edauk.com, website: www.edauk.com

Fellowship of Depressives Anonymous
Box FDA, Self Help Nottingham, Ormiston House,
32-36 Pelham Street, Nottingham NG1 2EG,
tel: 0870 774 4320, website: www.depressionanon.co.uk
A self-help organisation.

MDF – The Bipolar Organisation
Castle Works, 21 St George's Road, London SE1 6ES,
tel: 08456 340 540, fax: 020 7793 2639,
email: mdf@mdf.org.uk, website: www.mdf.org.uk
Helps people affected by manic depression.

Mind (National Association for Mental Health)
Mind 15-19 Broadway, London E15 4BQ,
Mind*info*Line: 0845 766 0163, tel: 020 8519 2122,
fax: 020 8522 1725, email: contact@mind.org.uk,
website: www.mind.org.uk

Mind Cymru, 3rd Floor, Quebec House, Castlebridge,
5-19 Cowbridge Road East, Cardiff CF11 9AB,
tel: 029 2039 5123, fax: 029 2034 6585

Rural Minds c/o South Staffs CVS,
1 Stafford Street, Brewood, Staffs ST19 9DX,
tel: 024 7641 4366, fax: 024 7641 4369,
email: ruralminds@ruralnet.org.uk

Mind has a network of over 200 local Mind associations throughout England and Wales. These offer supported housing, crisis helplines, drop-in centres, counselling, befriending, advocacy, employment and training schemes, and other services. To find contact details for your local association visit www.mind.org.uk/Mind+in+your+area

Rethink
28 Castle Street, Kingston upon Thames KT1 1SS, advice line: 020 8974 6814, tel: 0845 456 0455, email: info@rethink.org, website: www.rethink.org
Helps those affected by severe mental illness.

Samaritans
helpline: 08457 90 90 90, email: Jo@samaritans.org, website: www.samaritans.org
24-hour telephone helpline.

Saneline
1st Floor Cityside House, 40 Adler Street, London E1 1EE, Saneline: 0845 767 8000 (Mon-Fri 12 noon-11pm, Sat and Sun 12 noon-6pm), tel: 020 7375 1002, fax: 020 7375 2162, website: www.sane.org.uk
Saneline is a national out-of-hours telephone helpline providing information and support for anyone affected by mental health problems, including families and carers.

Body and mind

Alcoholics Anonymous (AA)
PO Box 1, Stonebow House, Stonebow, York YO1 7NJ,
helpline: 0845 769 7555, tel: 01904 644 026,
website: www.alcoholics-anonymous.org.uk

ASH (Action on Smoking and Health)
102 Clifton Street, London EC2A 4HW,
tel: 020 7739 5902, fax: 020 7613 0531,
email: enquiries@ash.org.uk, website: www.ash.org.uk

Quit
211 Old Street, London EC1V 9NR,
helpline: 0800 002 200, helpline email:
stopsmoking@quit.org.uk, tel: 020 7251 1551,
fax: 020 7251 1661, email: info@quit.org.uk,
website: www.quit.org.uk
Advice and support to stop smoking.

Weight Concern
Brook House, 2-16 Torrington Place, London WC1E 7HN,
tel: 0207 679 6636, fax: 020 7813 2848,
email: enquiries@weightconcern.org.uk,
website: www.weightconcern.org.uk

Employment

Acas
helpline: 08457 474 747 (Mon-Fri 8am-6pm), impaired hearing: 08456 061 600, website: www.acas.org.uk
Acas provides up-to-date information and independent advice on employment relations, working with employers and employees to solve problems.

Citizens Advice Bureau
website: www.citizensadvice.org.uk

Employment Tribunals
enquiry line: 0845 795 9775, minicom: 08457 573 722, website: www.employmenttribunals.gov.uk
Employment Tribunals are judicial bodies set up to resolve disputes over employment rights.

learndirect
helpline: 0800 101 900 website: www.learndirect.co.uk
Advice on courses and training.

WorkSMART
website: www.worksmart.org.uk
Helping working people get the best out of the world of work.

The elderly

Age Concern Cymru
Ty John Pathy, 13-14 Neptune Court, Vanguard Way,
Cardiff CF24 5PJ, tel: 029 2043 1555, fax: 029 2047 1418,
email: enquiries@accymru.org.uk,
website: www.accymru.org.uk

Age Concern England
Astral House, 1268 London Road, London SW16 4ER,
helpline: 0800 009 966, tel: 020 8765 7200,
fax: 020 8765 7211, website: www.ageconcern.org.uk

Alzheimer's Society
Gordon House, 10 Greencoat Place, London SW1P 1PH,
helpline: 0845 300 0336 (Mon-Fri 8.30am-6.30pm),
tel: 020 7306 0606, fax: 020 7306 0808,
email: enquiries@alzheimers.org.uk,
website:www.alzheimers.org.uk

Help the Aged
207-221 Pentonville Rd, London N1 9UZ,
helpline: 0808 800 6565, tel: 020 7278 1114,
fax: 020 7278 1116, email: info@helptheaged.org.uk,
website: www.helptheaged.org.uk

Parents

Association for Post-Natal Illness
145 Dawes Road, London SW6 7EB,
helpline: 020 7386 0868, fax: 020 7386 8885,
email: info@apni.org, website: www.apni.org

Parentline Plus
helpline: 0808 800 2222, textphone: 0800 783 6783,
tel: 020 7284 5500, fax: 020 7284 5501,
email: centraloffice@parentlineplus.org.uk,
website: www.parentlineplus.org.uk
Charity supporting anyone parenting a child.

SureStart
website: www.surestart.gov.uk
Government programme to deliver the best start in life
for every child.

YoungMinds
48-50 St John Street, London EC1M 4DG,
Parents' Information Service: 0800 018 2138 (Mon and
Fri 10am-1pm, Tues, Wed and Thurs 1-4pm, Wed 6-8pm),
email: enquiries@youngminds.org.uk,
website: www.youngminds.org.uk
Parents' Information Service offers support to people
coping with emotional and mental health problems
affecting their children and teenagers.

Relationships

National Family Mediation
7 The Close, Exeter EX1 1EZ, tel: 01392 271 610,
fax: 01392 271 945, email: general@nfm.org.uk,
website: www.nfm.u-net.com
Network of family mediation services.

Relate
Herbert Gray College, Little Church Street,
Rugby CV21 3AP, helpline: 0845 130 4010,
tel: 01788 573 241, email: enquiries@relate.org.uk,
website: www.relate.org.uk
Relationship counselling, mediation and support.

Treatments

British Association for Counselling and Psychotherapy (BACP)
BACP House, 35-37 Albert Street, Rugby CV21 2SG,
tel: 0870 443 5252, email: bacp@bacp.co.uk,
website: www.bacp.co.uk
See website or send A5 SAE for details of local
practitioners.

British Psychoanalytic Council
West Hill House, 6 Swains Lane, London N6 6QS,
tel: 020 7267 3626, fax: 020 7267 4772,
email: mail@pyschoanalytic-council.org,
website: www.psychoanalytic-council.org
A linking body of psychoanalytical psychotherapist
societies.

NHS Direct
helpline: 0845 4647, textphone: 0845 606 4647,
website: www.nhsdirect.nhs.uk

NICE (National Institute for Health and Clinical Excellence)
MidCity Place, 71 High Holborn, London WC1V 6NA,
tel: 020 7067 5800, fax: 020 7067 5801,
website: www.nice.org.uk
Contact for copies of guidelines for doctors and medical staff on caring for people with depression.

Thyromind
www.thyromind.info information on thyroid disease and mental illness.

UK Council for Psychotherapy (UKCP)
2nd Floor Edward House, 2 Wakley Street,
London EC1V 7LT, tel: 020 7014 9955,
email: info@psychotherapy.org.uk,
website: www.psychotherapy.org.uk
Umbrella organisation for psychotherapy in the UK. Maintains a voluntary register of qualified psychotherapists.

Young people

Childline
helpline: 0800 1111, website: www.childline.org.uk

Connexions Direct
helpline: 080 800 13219 (8am-2pm),
website: www.connexions-direct.com
Connexions Direct is a confidential service providing
information and advice to people aged 13-19.

Further reading

Beyond Prozac: healing mental distress without drugs, T. Lynch (PCCS Books 2004)

Climbing out of depression, S. Atkinson (Lion Publishing 1993)

Coping with anxiety and depression, S. Trickett (Sheldon 1997)

Depression: the way out of your prison (3rd ed), D. Rowe (Routledge 2003)

How to cope as a carer (Mind 2003)

How to help someone who is suicidal (Mind 2004)

How to improve your mental wellbeing (Mind 2006)

How to look after yourself (Mind 2004)

Making sense of antidepressants (Mind 2006)

Making sense of cognitive behaviour therapy (Mind 2004)

Making sense of counselling (Mind 2004)

Making sense of ECT (Mind 2003)

Making sense of psychotherapy and psychoanalysis (Mind 2004)

The Mind guide to physical activity (Mind 2004)

Mind rights guide 1: civil admission to hospital (Mind 2004)

The noonday demon: an anatomy of depression, A. Solomon (Random House 2001)

Overcoming depression, W. Dryden, S. Opie (Sheldon Press 2003)

Overcoming depression: a self-help guide using cognitive behavioural techniques, P. Gilbert (Constable 2000)

Sunbathing in the rain: a cheerful book about depression, G. Lewis (Flamingo 2003)

Understanding anxiety (Mind 2005)

Understanding bereavement (Mind 2005)

Understanding dual diagnosis (Mind 2004)

Understanding manic depression (bipolar disorder) (Mind 2003)

Understanding postnatal depression (Mind 2006)

Understanding seasonal affective disorder (Mind 2004)

Understanding the psychological effects of street drugs (Mind 2004)

When someone you love has depression, B. Baker
(Sheldon Press 2003)

To order any of these titles, or for a catalogue of
publications from Mind, send an A4 SAE to:

Mind Publications
15-19 Broadway
London E15 4BQ

T: 0844 448 4448
F: 020 8534 6399
e: publications@mind.org.uk
web: www.mind.org.uk

Visit the online shop to see details of all the publications
stocked.

Moving on from depression

Index